PERMING AND STRAIGHTENING
A Salon Handbook

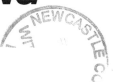

Other books of interest

COLOURING
A Salon Handbook
Lesley Hatton, Phillip Hatton and Alisoun Powell
0 632 01922 0

HYGIENE
A Salon Handbook
Second Edition
Phillip Hatton
0 632 02815 7

CUTTING AND STYLING
A Salon Handbook
Lesley Hatton and Phillip Hatton
0 632 01851 8

FOUNDATION HAIRDRESSING
Lesley Hatton and Phillip Hatton
0 632 02613 8

AFRO HAIR
A Salon Handbook
Phillip Hatton
0 632 02285 X

HAIRDRESSING BUSINESS MANAGEMENT
A Salon Handbook
Annette Mieske
0 632 02592 1

PERMING AND STRAIGHTENING
A Salon Handbook

Second Edition

Lesley Hatton
Phillip Hatton
BSc (Hons), DipEdMan, MIBiol, CBiol, MIT, FRIPHH, PGCE

OXFORD

BLACKWELL SCIENTIFIC PUBLICATIONS

LONDON EDINBURGH BOSTON
MELBOURNE PARIS BERLIN VIENNA

Copyright © Lesley Hatton, Phillip Hatton 1987, 1993

Blackwell Scientific Publications
Editorial Offices:
Osney Mead, Oxford OX2 0EL
25 John Street, London WC1N 2BL
23 Ainslie Place, Edinburgh EH3 6AJ
238 Main Street, Cambridge,
  Massachusetts 02142, USA
54 University Street, Carlton
  Victoria 3053, Australia

  Other Editorial Offices:
  Librairie Arnette SA
  2, rue Casimir-Delavigne
  75006 Paris
  France

  Blackwell Wissenschafts-Verlag GmbH
  Düsseldorfer Str. 38
  D-10707 Berlin
  Germany

  Blackwell MZV
  Feldgasse 13
  A-1238 Wien
  Austria

First published 1987
Reprinted 1989
Second edition 1993

Printed and bound in Great Britain by
the Alden Press, Oxford

DISTRIBUTORS

Marston Book Services Ltd
PO Box 87
Oxford OX2 0DT
(Orders: Tel: 0865 791155
        Fax: 0865 791927
        Telex: 837515)

USA
Blackwell Scientific Publications, Inc.
238 Main Street
Cambridge, MA 02142
(Orders: Tel: 800 759-6102
        617 876-7000)

Canada
Oxford University Press
70 Wynford Drive
Don Mills
Ontario M3C 1J9
(Orders: Tel: 416 441-2941)

Australia
Blackwell Scientific Publications Pty Ltd
54 University Street
Carlton, Victoria 3053
(Orders: Tel: 03 347-5552)

British Library
Cataloguing in Publication Data

A catalogue record for this book is
available from the British Library

ISBN 0-632-03316-9

Library of Congress
Cataloging in Publication Data

Hatton, Lesley.
    Perming and straightening: a salon
  handbook/Lesley Hatton, Phillip Hatton.
  — 2nd ed.
      p.   cm.
    Includes index.
    ISBN 0-632-03316-9
    1. Permanent waving.   2. Hair—Relaxing.
  I. Hatton, Phillip.   II. Title.
  TT972.H37   1992
  646.7'242—dc20   92-15847
                                    CIP

Dedication

In memory of our fathers – Walter Ralph (L.H.)
                    – John Hatton (P.H.)

Contents

About This Book

This book has been written for everyone who perms and straightens hair in salons. You may be an experienced hairdresser, or a beginner training in a salon, school or college. If you digest the information carefully, it will make you a more knowledgeable hairdresser.

Poor results in the salon are almost always blamed on the client's hair! If you do not get the result that you wanted it is because something wrong has been *done*. It could be the choice of product, its strength, processing time, the technique used, or indeed, the hair itself. Correct preparation, including a discussion with the client and testing the hair as necessary, will ensure good results and happy customers!

This book is different from others that deal with perming and straightening because it answers the questions that you will ask. It contains the scientific background, as well as the practical know-how of perming and straightening hair. Everything is set out in a down-to-earth way, with no mysterious jargon. Diagrams have been included to explain how the various chemicals which are used actually work. The differences between the various products, and how they are meant to be used will become apparent. Safety is emphasised throughout the book, but precautions are only given if there are reasons for them. The fashion techniques include clear photographs to help you achieve what has been explained.

If you are training hairdressers, or are still learning yourself, the questions at the end of each chapter will prove invaluable. They will take you through each chapter, step-by-step, until you have a thorough knowledge of perming and straightening hair.

Afro hair has been dealt with in this book in a clear and concise way. We hope that this will clear away the mystery that surrounds Afro hair. Don't be frightened of it, hair is hair! (For more information, please refer to *Afro Hair* by Phillip Hatton.)

Keep the book in the salon so that you can refer to it as necessary. You (or your staff) will have access to the information needed, written specifically for hairdressers, by people who really know, and care, about hair.

Acknowledgements

We would like to thank the following people for their contributions to the writing of this book:

Kevin and Maureen Bura
Clynol Hair
Goldwell (Hair Cosmetics) Ltd
L'Oréal
Joan Newton of Redken Laboratories Ltd
Kathy Brown of Wella (GB) Ltd
Zotos (UK) Ltd

Note: Although the term 'curler' has been used throughout this book, the equivalent North American term is 'rod'.

Lesley Hatton
Phillip Hatton

PUBLISHER'S NOTE

It is extremely important that anyone working with relaxers is trained to realise that there is a difference in the way that active ingredients work. For this reason there should be no intermixing of products from different ranges unless hairdressers are absolutely certain of what they are doing. There have been legal actions where it was obvious that hairdressers had not followed manufacturers' instructions. Also, if you are doing a COSHH assessment for your salon (something that salon owners/managers are responsible for), ammonium thioglycollate 'relaxers' should be referred to as *straighteners*. This fulfils the Health and Safety Executive definition.

1
Basic Facts

1.1   Hair facts

What is hair?

Hair is composed of a type of protein, called keratin, which is different from other proteins because it contains sulphur. It is this sulphur that allows us to perm and straighten hair. Keratin is also a major constituent of our skin and nails, therefore hairdressing chemicals affect them as well as the hair for which they were intended. This is why you should take care to protect your hands when using hairdressing products.

Hair can be classified into types. *Lanugo* hair is found on the human foetus before birth, usually as an unpigmented coat of fine, soft hair. It is shed between the seventh and eighth month of the pregnancy – so we can now ignore it as far as hairdressing goes. *Vellus* hair is the fine downy hair found on the body and, if this is dark, some women find it embarrassing (on the arms, legs, or upper lip) because they regard it as a masculine characteristic. If it is bleached, using a product designed for such hair, it becomes much less noticeable. The hair we as hairdressers are concerned with, however, is called *terminal* hair. It is coarser and is found on the scalp, on men's faces, under the arms, and on the pubic area. The growth and distribution of terminal facial and body hair is controlled by the male hormones – the *androgens* – which start to be secreted at puberty in both men and women (though more so in men).

Unfortunately, a number of women have trouble as they get older, with facial hairs becoming coarser. This is caused by hormonal changes, and if the hair is unsightly it is best to have it removed by electrolysis. (This may require several treatments.)

How does a hair grow?

A hair grows from a minute pit in the skin called a *hair follicle*. The hair that we see emerging from the scalp is dead, but at the base of the follicle the hair is alive and actively growing. As the hair we see is dead, we cannot alter how it grows by any hairdressing process or treatment. Cutting does not alter the speed of growth or the diameter of the hair. Thus the story that shaving legs makes the hairs grow coarser is untrue. Many young men who shave for the first time are convinced that shaving has made their beards coarser, but it is only because recently shaved stubble feels coarser than a beard which has been left to grow. The saying that regular haircuts make your hair grow faster is also untrue.

Once a hair has been damaged, it cannot be permanently repaired. It is possible to mask the damage with special conditioners, but the only way to change the quality of the hair permanently is through correct care and diet, since food and oxygen get into the hair through the blood supply.

This is why the hairdresser must be fully aware of the potential damage that can be caused to hair by the various hairdressing chemicals and treatments that are used. Adjusting curl is probably the most technically complicated thing that one can do to hair. Clients see the hairdresser as a professional person who knows what he or she is doing and knows what is best for their hair. Make sure that their faith is properly placed.

What is the structure of a hair like?

Figure 1.1 shows a highly magnified hair. The photograph was taken with an electron microscope and what you are seeing is a hair magnified over one thousand times. The scales that you can see are one of several layers (about seven in European hair, and up to eleven in Chinese hair). This outer layer is known as the *cuticle*. There are more cuticle layers around

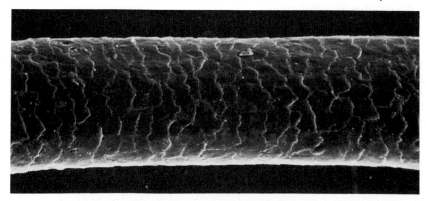

Fig. 1.1 Electron micrograph of a hair showing the layers of cuticle overlapping each other (× 1100).

the hair shaft near the base of the hair than there are towards the older tip of the hair, purely because of wear and tear. It is the protective layer of the hair and prevents things from entering the layers below. The cuticle is rather like the tiles on a roof which protect a house from the weather. But, unlike a roof, there are several layers. The free ends of the overlapping scales (called imbrications) point upwards in the direction of the hair growth, that is, towards the tip. If you take a hair between the finger and thumb and gently rub it up and down the hair, you will find it feels smooth from root to point, but rough from point to root. This is because of the tips of the cuticle scales causing resistance. Because the cuticle scales are translucent (allowing some light to pass through them) we can see the colour of the hair in the layer below.

If the cuticle is damaged by excessive physical or chemical treatment, the second layer of the hair, the *cortex*, may be exposed to injury. This second layer forms the bulk of the hair and it is in this part that the chemical changes of perming and straightening take place. Figure 1.2 shows these cortical cells clearly.

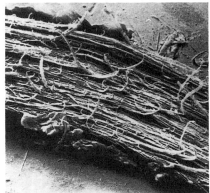

Fig. 1.2 Electron micrograph of a hair which has been cut through its centre to reveal the strand-like cortical cells of the hair (reproduced courtesy of Wella).

The cortex is the most important layer of the hair and makes up 75 to 90 per cent of the hair's bulk. It contains the natural pigment of the hair (mostly melanin if the hair is black to brown or mostly pheomelanin if the hair is yellow to red). This pigment is produced at the bottom of the follicle by a cell called a melanocyte. Many of the physical properties of hair are dependent on the cortex. These include:

- Strength
- Elasticity
- Direction and type of growth (straight, curly)
- Diameter of hair shaft

Put simply, the cortex has a structure rather like a bunch of straws (called macrofibrils) which are held together by a network of keratin fibres. Within each of the 'straws' are finer tubes (called microfibrils), which contain a group of three coiled polypeptide chains (known as the

Cross-linkages of hair

There are three types of cross-linkage in the keratin of hair, illustrated in Figure 1.4:

(1) *Disulphide bonds*
These are the most important bonds as far as perming and straightening are concerned as it is these that are broken to allow the alteration of the hair shape. The amino acid cystine forms a link through its central disulphide bond between two adjacent polypeptide chains. It is this cystine or disulphide linkage that we were referring to earlier when we said that the linkages were like rungs of a ladder. They are very strong bonds which are broken only by chemicals.

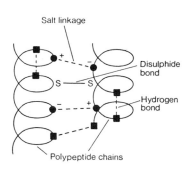

Fig. 1.4 The different cross-linkages of hair. The most important of these are the disulphide bonds because they maintain the structure of the hair and are difficult to break. The hydrogen bonds and salt linkages are much weaker but there are more of them. Hydrogen bonds are broken during setting but are easily reformed.

Not all the sulphur in hair is taken up by cystine linkages, as most hairdressers believe. There are free sulphurs on some polypeptides which are not opposite other sulphurs, so they cannot form disulphide bonds. Where this occurs, the amino acid is called cysteine (note the spelling!).

Most hair contains between 4–5 per cent sulphur, but natural red hair may contain up to 8 per cent sulphur. Because this is about twice as much as normal hair, red hair, with its higher sulphur content, is more resistant and difficult to treat.

(2) *Salt linkages*
The amino acids that form polypeptides may have free acid (negative) or basic amino (positive) groups. If a free negative in one polypeptide chain lies opposite a free positive in an adjacent chain there will be an attraction between them. Opposite electrical charges attract, rather like the North and South poles of magnets. These salt linkages are also called ionic or electrostatic bonds. Because they are weaker than the disulphide linkages they can be easily broken by weak acids or alkalis. If you quickly run a nylon comb through your hair for a minute it will be able to attract and

pick up a small piece of paper. The comb has picked up an electrostatic charge from the hair and the opposite charge induced in the piece of paper attracts the two together.

(3) *Hydrogen bonds*

These weak bonds are due to the attraction between hydrogen atoms and oxygen atoms (like the salt linkages, this is an electrostatic attraction). This bonding can occur in a polypeptide chain (between the coils), or between adjacent polypeptide chains. Since they form cross-bonds, they help the disulphide bonds to keep adjacent polypeptide chains together, giving 'body' to the hair. Although the hydrogen bonds are very weak, many more of them are present than any other bond in the hair. Hydrogen bonds can be broken by water and most weak chemicals.

Free amino acids

Between the chains of keratin in the cortex of the hair are found 'free' amino acids. These do not appear to play any structural role but help to hold moisture within the cortex. The level of moisture is maintained at about 10 per cent by the amino acids and the coating of sebum on the cuticle. Moisture is important to keep the hair pliable.

In hair where the cuticle is damaged, shampooing can remove some of the free amino acids. The level of moisture in the cortex falls and the condition of the hair suffers. To counteract this some treatments contain free amino acids or treated protein.

1.3 Skin facts

What is the skin?

Skin is the outside covering of the body. It has an average area of 18 square feet and an average weight of 6 pounds or 3 kilograms. It is remarkably complex and will be looked at here in outline.

Figure 1.5 shows a generalised vertical section of skin. This is a diagram that includes all relevant skin structures, although some would not be found on particular parts of the body (have you got hair on the palms of your hands?).

What do the parts of the skin do?

Briefly, the skin is a protective layer with numerous nerve endings which can respond to heat, cold, pain, pressure and touch. If we get either too

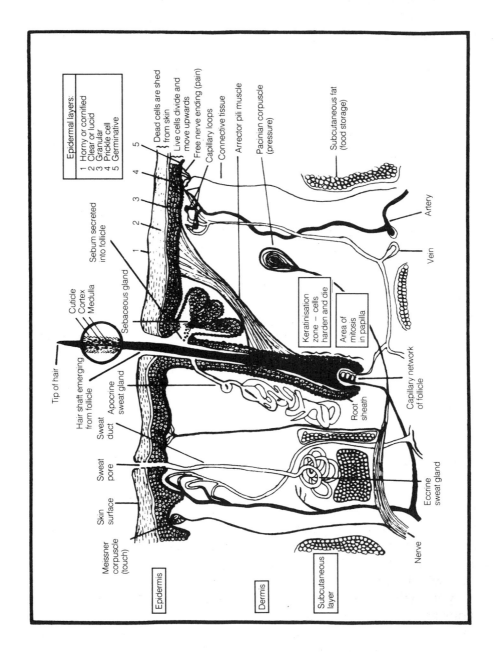

Fig. 1.5 Vertical section of the skin.

hot or too cold the skin can help us reach normal body temperature again. It stores food in the form of fat (something that many of us know to our cost!), and can manufacture vitamin D (needed to absorb calcium from our food for healthy bones and teeth) and melanin (needed to protect live skin cells from being burnt by the sun's ultraviolet rays which could otherwise cause scarring or even cancer).

Hair follicles are found almost everywhere (but not on the palms of hands, soles of feet or the lips). The sebaceous glands, which are attached to the follicle, secrete an oily liquid called sebum. This helps to waterproof and lubricate the skin, as well as helping to prevent fungal infections such as ringworm. The hair is also coated with sebum and this helps to maintain moisture in the cortex of the hair. Sebaceous glands are under the control of hormones (particularly the male hormones, androgens) which make the glands enlarge and secrete more at puberty. Acne and greasy skin is directly related to this. On the hairs of the underarms, the follicles also have a special type of sweat gland, the apocrine sweat gland. These secrete a sweat which is mostly water but also contains fatty acids which create body odour when they are broken down by bacteria. The hair follicle also has an arrector pili muscle which makes the hair stand on end. This is supposed to trap a layer of warm air around the body but would only be really effective on extremely hairy people.

The normal sweat gland (eccrine sweat gland) produces sweat, which is mostly water with a little salt. This sweat cools the skin when it evaporates. It is under the control of the nerves, as most of us have found when we have been nervous and had sweaty palms. In hot climates loss of sweat without drinking can result in dehydration.

The epidermis is the top layer of the skin. The lower cells are alive, dividing by *mitosis* (this is the type of cell division where a cell splits in two and produces two exact copies of itself) and pushing upwards where they become full of keratin and die. When this process happens too quickly, *pityriasis* (dandruff) results (this can happen anywhere on the body and not just on the scalp). The epidermis is protective, and contains no nerves or blood vessels. Without the top horny layer, water loss would be increased by twenty times, which would mean possible death by dehydration. The hair follicle and sweat glands are actually part of the epidermis, which has down-growths into the dermis. If you look closely at Fig. 1.5 you will see that the germinative layer of the epidermis is continuous around the follicle and glands.

Because the sebum and sweat laying on the skin's surface have an acid pH, we say that the skin has an 'acid mantle'. This pH of between 4.5–5.5 discourages the growth of bacteria on the skin and also helps to keep the cuticle of the hair closed (see [1.4]).

Chemicals that we use on the hair in perming and straightening can be extremely caustic and can either irritate the skin causing an allergic reaction (dermatitis) or burn it. A chemical burn can cause permanent skin damage. It could result in hair loss in that area and loss of feeling if nerve cells are destroyed.

1.4   pH

What is pH?

The term 'pH' is simply a way of expressing how acid or alkaline something is, on a scale from 0 to 14. 7.0, in the middle, is the neutral point, and indicates when something is neither acid nor alkaline.

Acids contain hydrogen ions (positively charged hydrogen atoms). The stronger an acid is, the greater the concentration of hydrogen ions it contains. A pH of below 7.0 is acid; the smaller the number, the stronger the acid. A pH of 2 is a stronger acid than 3, and 0 is the strongest acid.

Alkalis contain hydroxide ions (oxygen and hydrogen atoms joined together with a negative charge). The stronger an alkali is, the more hydroxide ions it contains. A pH above 7.0 is alkaline; the larger the number, the stronger the alkali. A pH of 10 is a stronger alkali than 8, and 14 is the strongest alkali.

Water is neutral in pH (i.e. pH = 7) because it contains the same number of hydrogen ions as hydroxide ions.

$$H_2O \longrightarrow H^+ + OH^-$$

water gives hydrogen hydroxide
ion   ion

Remember, if a solution contained more hydrogen than hydroxide ions it would be acid, and alkaline if it contained more hydroxide than hydrogen ions. Also, if 7.0 is neutral (neither acid nor alkaline), the nearer a number is to 7.0 the weaker an acid or alkali is.

How do I test pH?

If you look at Fig. 1.6, which shows how hairdressing chemicals affect the hair, you will see two ways of testing pH. One is litmus, a dye which becomes red in acids and blue in alkalis. This is available as paper or a liquid. It has the disadvantage that it can only tell you if a chemical is acid or alkaline, not how weak or strong it is. The second product is called universal indicator paper, and this changes over a range of colours which correspond to different pHs. The colour is simply matched up to a chart.

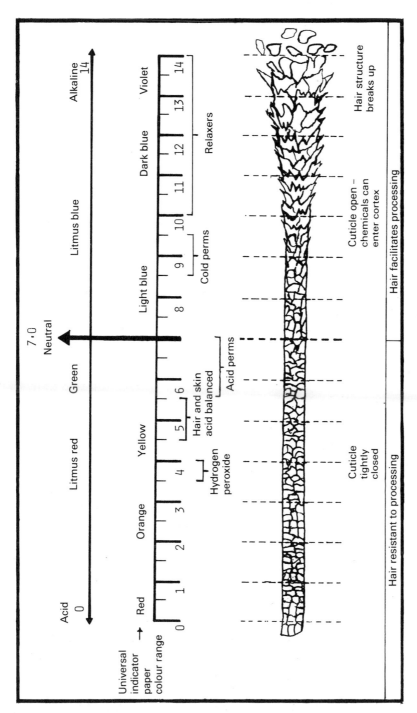

Fig. 1.6 pH chart showing how hairdressing chemicals affect the hair.

Again, this is available as paper or liquid. When the product manufacturers make their various products they use delicate electronic pH meters to make sure that the pH is correct.

Why is pH important to hairdressing?

pH is important for a number of reasons. Acids close the cuticle of hair, making it reflect light and appear shiny (remember the *c* in acid for *close*). The cuticle is closed tightly so will resist chemical processing, as the chemicals cannot pass through the cuticle into the cortex.

Alkalis open the cuticle, making the hair appear dull as light is scattered rather than being uniformly reflected. Many hairdressing chemicals are alkaline because they will open the cuticle and allow the chemical to enter the cortex. Porous hair with its open cuticle will thus facilitate processing. This is why perm lotions are available in different strengths, because very porous hair might process too quickly.

Alkalis cause the hair to swell up. A strong alkali can therefore cause more damage than a strong acid because it gets into the cortex easily (whereas the acid closes the cuticle and so cannot enter the cortex very quickly). From Fig. 1.6 it can be seen how the hair swells and eventually breaks up. Chemicals that destroy hair are called depilatories, which are alkaline and work by swelling the cortex to facilitate entry into it. In the cortex a depilatory breaks down the peptide bonds of the hair. (The hydrolysed keratin found in conditioners consists of small pieces of keratin which have been broken down in this way. Their small size allows entry into the cortex of the hair.)

To counteract damage to the hair when we use alkaline chemicals, we often use acid rinses afterwards. These close the cuticle and neutralise any remaining alkaline chemicals in the hair.

Acid-balanced products have the same pH as the hair and skin – which have a pH of 4.5 to 5.5, average 5.4 – and so do not upset the natural pH.

1.5   Curly and straight hair

Before beginning an investigation of the techniques used to perm and straighten hair it is worth considering why hair is naturally straight or curly.

Why do some people have curly hair?

Without looking at what is actually going on at the base of the hair follicle there are a number of factors that determine whether or not someone has curly hair. Heredity has a major influence. If your parents both have curly hair it is likely that you will as well. If one of your grandparents had curly hair but your parents did not, it is likely you would have straight hair, but there would still be a chance of curls. Hair of Negro origin is characteristically very tightly curled while hair of Chinese origin is characteristically straight.

Diet cannot cause hair to be curly, but it can cause naturally curly hair to lose its waves. The diet would have to be lacking proteins derived from amino acids which contain sulphur. This is more likely to happen to young mothers who need extra protein or older people who have changed their diet.

Illness can also cause a loss of curl as hair growth often suffers. During convalescence after an illness there is often a slow return of natural curl.

How does the hair get its curl?

Many textbooks have claimed that the shapes of the hair shaft and follicle determine whether or not a hair is straight or curly.

Some believed that a hair follicle with a circular cross-section generated a straight hair while a follicle with an oval cross-section generated a curved hair. However, this theory is wrong since it is now known that not all round hairs are straight or all flattened hairs curly.

The other popular but mistaken theory, is that the shape of the hair follicle determines the natural curl of the hair. This theory relies on the fact that hair cells are soft and therefore 'pliable' when first produced, only becoming completely keratinised or hardened as they pass up the follicle to the skin surface. If these cells harden in a straight follicle, it was thought that the hair would also be straight. Conversely, if they harden in a curved follicle, it was thought that the hair would be wavy or curly. This theory does not account for changes in curl which were mentioned above (diet, age, motherhood and illness). The follicle is very small so it cannot be the only reason. Otherwise Negroid hair, which has a very tight curl formation, would simply come out from the skin and curl straight back over into the skin.

The secret of natural curl formation actually lies in actual cell division in the dermal papilla of the hair.

How does cell division determine curl?

Basically, if you think of the base of a hair follicle as a circular clock, and all the cells at each number are dividing at the same rate, the resultant hair

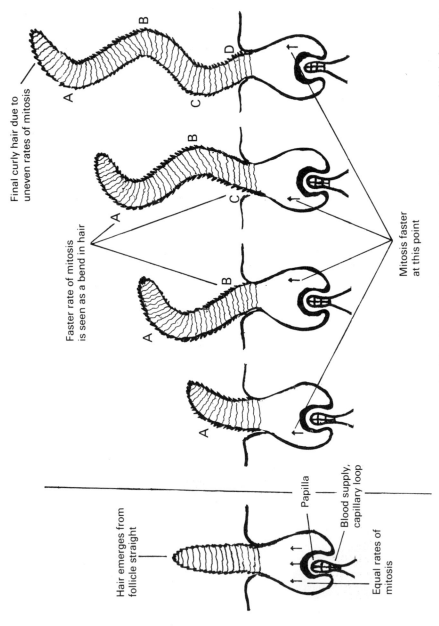

Fig. 1.7   Cyclical theory of hair growth. The first hair has emerged straight from the follicle because the rates of mitosis in the papilla are identical. However, the second hair has emerged curly because the rate of mitosis has not been even. The hair bends over to the opposite side where cell division is fastest.

produced will be straight. But what would happen if the cells at 3 o'clock began to divide faster than the rest of the cells? The hair would not grow straight, but would bend over towards 9 on the clock. If the cell division at 3 o'clock then slowed down, while the cell division at 9 o'clock increased, the hair would now bend towards 3 on the clock. Figure 1.7 shows how the natural curl may be formed in a hair according to this cyclical theory of hair growth, the degree of curl depending on how quickly this uneven rate of cell division shifts from one side of the germinal matrix of the papilla to the other. This is the only theory of hair growth that really accounts for the tight curls of Afro hair.

Is there any difference in structure between curly and straight hair?

Modern technology has shown us that there is a difference in structure between curly and straight hair. In curly hair there is a difference in structure between one side of a hair compared with the other. This gives rise to two different types of cortex, an 'ortho' and a 'para' cortex. This dual cortex has been shown by microscopical staining techniques. The ortho cortex (see Fig. 1.8) has a less dense structure and a lower sulphur content than the para cortex and always lies on the outside of the wave.

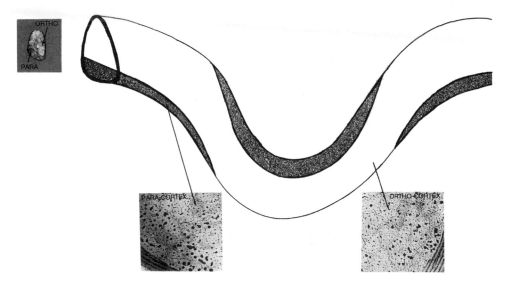

Fig. 1.8   The ortho and para cortex of a curly black hair, note the shape of the cross-section of hair. The separate cortexes can only be seen clearly in black hair with a high degree of curl. (This diagram has been adapted with the permission of Wella.)

The structure is comparable with European hair which has been permanently waved; the hair on the outer curve is stretched (and therefore less dense) while the hair on the inner curve is compressed (and is therefore more dense). Only the cyclical theory of hair growth explains this.

Many Afro hairdressers talk of the hair having 'more keratin'. What they are, in fact, referring to is the higher sulphur content of the para cortex.

1.6   Questions

1   What is hair composed of?
2   Why should you protect your hands when perming?
3   What is lanugo hair?
4   What is vellus hair?
5   What is terminal hair?
6   Where does the hair grow from?
7   Does cutting hair make it grow faster?
8   How can you improve the condition of hair permanently?
9   Describe the outer layer of the hair.
10   How could you tell the difference between European and Chinese hair by looking at the cuticle?
11   What does translucent mean?
12   Describe the cortex of the hair.
13   What is a melanocyte?
14   Is the medulla important to hairdressing processes?
15   What elements are found in keratin?
16   Describe the three types of bonds or linkages found in hair.
17   Which bond is the most important to perming?
18   Why are the free amino acids in hair important?
19   Does all skin have hair follicles present?
20   Describe the three types of gland found in the skin.
21   What does the arrector pili muscle do?
22   What is mitosis?
23   Is dandruff found only on the scalp?
24   Why is the pH of the skin slightly acid?
25   What is pH a measurement of?
26   What does a pH of 7.0 signify?
27   How could you test the pH of a hairdressing chemical?
28   Why are many hairdressing chemicals alkaline?
29   What is the real reason for the curl in hair?
30   What are the two types of cortex?
31   Which type of cortex would be found on the inside curve of a curl?

2

Take Precautions!

You are responsible for the safety and well-being of your client. Many of the chemicals used in perming and relaxing are potentially very dangerous, so it is important to minimise risks by taking the necessary precautions and carrying out appropriate tests. It is possible for you to burn a client's skin and leave permanent scars, or cause a client's hair to break off, or even cause a client to lose his or her sight, *and you would be responsible.* Any of these disasters could happen if you do not take care. You could be sued by the client and if it were not settled outside the courts you might get some very undesirable publicity in the local newspapers!

It is important to remember that clients are not always aware of the products they have on their hair, or of the significance of answering your questions truthfully. We have all come across the client who has a regrowth and insists that her hair is natural and has never been tinted! Unfortunately for the hairdresser, not all products used previously on the hair are as obvious to detect as this.

When perming or relaxing hair, get into good working habits. Eventually you will do things automatically. Tell your client what you are doing and why. They will appreciate your care and professionalism.

2.1 Examining the scalp

Before commencing any chemical work on the hair, an examination of the scalp must first be made. This examination must be positive and thorough, but not embarrassing for the client. It is best carried out during your initial talk with the client, while you discuss the intended style.

Why should the scalp be examined?

Firstly, the scalp must always be examined in case any infectious conditions are present, such as impetigo or ringworm. In general, look for pustules or areas of redness. If the scalp has been scratched a lot, particularly in the nape region and just above the ears, check there for the presence of lice. Do not expect to see lice moving about! Check carefully for the eggs of the lice, called nits, which would be cemented to the hairshaft within a centimetre or so (half an inch) of the scalp. If nits are present (rather than flakes of dandruff), they cannot be removed with a comb. If anything infectious is found, *under no conditions offer the client a service*. You may have an angry client, depending on how tactfully you deal with the situation, but at least you are protecting your staff and other clientele from possible infection. If you can tell the client what is wrong, quietly with minimal fuss, and explain that you will welcome her back once it has been dealt with, she will probably appreciate the standard of your service. Do not deal with any infectious condition in the salon yourself, but refer the client to a doctor or trichologist, if necessary.

There are also a number of non-infectious scalp conditions which you might come across during an examination of the scalp. It is important to be able to recognise these as non-infectious in case you give offence to the client. Psoriasis can look unsightly and can easily be mistaken for an infectious condition. It is usually present as large silvery plaques of scale, which can be removed to reveal red areas underneath. Generally, clients will know if they have psoriasis. Perming and straightening can be performed as normal, provided that the skin is not broken – in fact, they can help to clear the scalp up temporarily! If your client has dandruff, it is simply the overproduction of skin scales, but could you sell them a good anti-dandruff treatment as an after-care service?

If there are any breaks in the skin surface, such as cuts or scratches, this could present problems. Perming or relaxing products coming into contact with an opening in the skin will cause severe discomfort and the skin will become inflamed. This could lead to problems such as dermatitis or scalp burns.

Work must never begin on hair without prior discussion between the hairdresser and client, however familiar you are with them. Scalp conditions can change suddenly, so always establish that the scalp is in good health.

For further reading on scalp conditions, see *Hygiene – A Salon Handbook*.

How should the scalp be examined?

Use a wide-toothed comb to divide the hair and examine all over the scalp.

You may ask the client if he or she is aware of any sores, cuts or itchy areas. Explain that these might be more sensitive to the chemicals that you will be using. Do not use a brush at this stage as the bristles may scratch the scalp.

What is the procedure if you find broken skin?

If you find an area of broken skin on the client's scalp it is recommended that the perm or relaxer treatment is postponed until it has healed. However, many hairdressers would proceed with treatment if the area of broken skin is small. The area should be protected with some barrier cream (such as vaseline or petroleum jelly) and the surrounding hair sectioned off so that it is not permed. The client will probably prefer this to having to wait until the scalp has healed. Always try to keep the lotion off the scalp.

2.2 *Assessing previous perming or relaxing treatment*

When we analyse a head of hair for perming or relaxing treatments the client may have already had such a service within the past few months. Clients will answer your questions about previous chemical treatment, but can you be sure that their answers are totally honest? Clients may feel too embarrassed to admit that they had previous treatment at another salon, or had a perm which did not last.

Why is it important to establish previous chemical treatment?

Once hair has been subjected to chemical processing from perms or relaxers, its internal structure becomes weaker and prone to further damage. Perming or relaxing hair which has undergone previous chemical treatment will be more likely to result in a weaker type of hair that will not retain moisture, and will be dry or 'like straw'. The damage may be so extensive that the hair will break off.

How can you establish previous chemical treatment?

Besides questioning the client, there are a number of ways by which you can establish previous chemical treatment.

On European (Caucasian) hair:
  A previous perm carried out four months ago may not be apparent when

the hair is dry, because the hair may have been set or blow-dried (which will stretch the hair out). It is therefore necessary to wet the hair to see whether permanent curl is present. Wetting hair will cause set or blow-dried hair (beta keratin) to return to its normal state (alpha keratin). For more on this, see *Cutting and Styling – A Salon Handbook*.

On Afro hair:

If a client comes to the salon for a regrowth relaxer treatment, you will probably be able to see the difference between the previously relaxed hair and the new hair growth quite distinctly. If the hair was permed before, this may be a little more difficult to establish. This is because the curl formation of Afro hair can sometimes be so strong that the permed hair will begin to revert back to its original, naturally curly state, over a period of months. In such a case, there is no need to shampoo the hair. Instead, massage a protective polymer product into the ends of the hair. This works on the same principle as a curl activator, releasing any curl in the hair, therefore defining the regrowth more clearly. Protective polymer products contain substances which moisturise the hair and coat it with a protective film of protein. This is penetrable by chemical products, and is similar to the pre-perm products used on European hair.

If previous chemical treatment is established, can you proceed with further chemical processing?

In most cases it is quite safe to proceed with further chemical treatment but you should carry out a thorough analysis and choose the product strength to suit the hair condition. There are also protecting products, such as pre-perm treatments and polymers which help to even out porosity and act as a buffer to the chemicals.

If the hair has previously been relaxed you will not be able to perm it successfully. Hair has only a certain number of disulphide bonds, and in relaxed hair this number will have been drastically reduced. To understand the chemistry of this, see Chapters 5 and 6.

It is possible to relax hair that has been previously permed, provided that you carry out the necessary analysis and protect the hair as required. A test curl will, of course, confirm whether or not the hair will perm successfully (see [2.7]).

2.3 Incompatibility test

What is an incompatibility test?

This test indicates whether or not any products previously used on the hair will react unfavourably with the products that you intend to use. It is specifically used to test for the presence of metallic salts which are contained in some hair colour preparations and could cause the hair to change colour, smoulder and even break off!

What types of colorant contain metallic salts?

Metallic salts are most commonly found in so-called 'hair colour restorers'. These are products which are used regularly over a period of time to give back colour to grey hair. On each application, the hair is coated with metallic salts (frequently lead) which subsequently react with the atmosphere to produce a dark colour. Because the colour takes time to develop it is referred to as a progressive colorant. The best-known product is *Grecian 2000*.

Some henna preparations also contain metallic salts, and these are usually referred to as being 'compound'. Their addition allows henna to have a greater colour range and lasting power.

Some temporary colours also contain metallic salts. These are usually available as spray colours (aerosols), gels or mousses, and frequently contain metallic glitter. For further information, see *Colouring – A Salon Handbook*.

How can you tell if metallic salts are present on the hair?

The surest way is to carry out an incompatibility test. You might suspect that metallic salts are on the hair because it has a greenish tinge to it, or because of the way it feels. Don't assume that clients will tell you if you ask them, as they may not want people to know they are grey and colour their hair. Older clients are most likely to use these preparations. If in doubt, carry out the test.

What do you need to carry out an incompatibility test?

glass container
20 volume hydrogen peroxide (6 per cent)
ammonia (0.880 ammonium hydroxide)
hair samples from client
sellotape
record card

How is an incompatibility test carried out?

- Prepare the hair samples by cutting from an unnoticeable area and secure at the root end with tape. Make sure your samples are from the areas you estimate to be most affected by the metallic salts. You may need more than one sample.
- Mix together twenty parts of the peroxide with one part of the ammonium hydroxide in the glass container. If ammonium hydroxide is not available in the salon, substitute perm lotion instead. Ammonium hydroxide will speed up any reaction that occurs; peroxide alone would be too slow.
- Immerse the sample(s) into the solution. Leave them in the solution for thirty minutes as some hair might be slow to react.
- Check the sample(s) for the presence of bubbles and feel the container to see if it has got any warmer. The hair might also change colour. If any of these occur it is *a positive reaction*.
- A positive reaction means that you cannot use any chemical that contains hydrogen peroxide on a client, as it will react violently and could damage both the hair and scalp.
- The metallic salts can also combine with the sulphur bonds in the cortex, interfering with perming or relaxing.

Can hair containing metallic salts be permed or relaxed?

The simple answer is an emphatic 'no'. Explain to the client that if you were to proceed with the perm or relaxer, his or her hair would be totally ruined and could even break off due to the adverse chemical reaction that would occur. Also, the scalp could be seriously burnt by the heat evolved by this reaction.

Claims have been made that the metallic salts can be stripped by special treatments, but these have proved unreliable. The only way to remove metallic dyes properly and completely is to let them grow out so that they can be cut off.

2.4   Porosity test

What is a porosity test?

A porosity test assesses the hair for external damage. That is, the degree of damage to the outside layer of the hair, the cuticle.

What does porosity mean?

Porosity describes the cuticle's ability to absorb moisture and hairdressing products. Porous hair will obviously allow products to penetrate more easily into the hair than will non-porous hair (see Fig. 2.1). The porosity of the hair will vary on different parts of the head and also on each individual strand of hair. The older a hair is, the more likely it will be that the ends of the hair are porous; it will have been subjected to more abuse such as from chemicals, drying or weathering (sun, sea and wind). This is why people with long hair find that the ends of their hair feel drier and rougher compared to the middle lengths or roots.

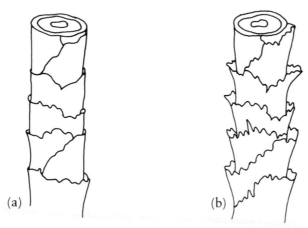

Fig. 2.1   (a) Non-porous and (b) porous hair.

What makes hair become porous?

Damage to the cuticle can be caused in two ways:

(a)   chemically
(b)   physically

Chemical damage is caused by hairdressing products which are alkaline, as these .ause the hair to swell and open up the cuticle (see [1.4]). This leaves the hair more susceptible to further damage, both internal and external. As so many hairdressing treatments involve alkaline chemicals, a certain amount of cuticle damage is unavoidable.

Physical damage can be caused in a number of ways. The regular use of heat is one of the most common. Many people use tongs, heated rollers, pressing combs, crimping irons or excessive heat from a hairdrier every day. Too much sunlight can also affect the cuticle. Back-combing, harsh brushing or the use of elastic bands can also cause damage. The ends of the hair, being the oldest part, will be most damaged.

How do you test for porosity?

Take a few strands of hair and hold firmly near the points. Slide your fingers down the hair shaft to the roots (against the lie of the cuticle). The rougher the hair feels, the more porous it is (see Fig. 2.2).

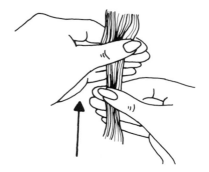

Fig. 2.2   Porosity test.

Remember that you may need to test several areas as porosity is never even and will vary over the whole head. The front hair will usually be more porous than the back because this is the area that receives more physical attention (brushing, etc.) and damage from the sun and wind as it is more exposed than the hair at the back.

Why should you test for porosity?

If the hair is porous, it means that the cuticle is open or has actually broken off, in varying degrees, along the hair's length. As the chemicals for perming and relaxing hair need to enter the cortex to work on the sulphur bonds, the chemicals will enter it at different speeds depending on the cuticle porosity. The hair which is most porous will allow penetration most quickly. The hair in such areas will have more air spaces and will therefore absorb more lotion. This will lead to more rapid processing here, and possible severe damage before the rest of the hair is processed. Results will be uneven with possible breakage.

Can the porosity of hair be improved?

The simple answer is 'yes', but only temporarily. Conditioners help to smooth the cuticle, coating the hair with a film which 'fills-in' the places where cuticle scales have actually been broken off. Acid rinses will close the cuticle scales and leave the hair less porous.

Can conditioners be used on porous hair before perming?

Many surface conditioners coat the hair with a film of wax or oil which would act as a barrier to the perm lotion passing into the cortex. Do not use normal conditioners before perming for this reason.

What can be used to even out porosity before perming?

Most manufacturers of perm products now produce 'pre-perm treatments' which are used before perming to even out the porosity of the hair. Although they work on the same principle as surface conditioners their special ingredients allow the perming products to pass through the cuticle. Many contain protein fillers which, as the name implies, fill in the most porous areas to equalise porosity along the hair shaft. Because the filler has similar chemical properties as the hair, it permits improved results with less damage.

How is a pre-perm treatment applied?

For the majority of perms, the hair is first shampooed and towel-dried. Pre-perm treatments are sprinkled directly from the bottle onto the hair. Combing the hair through will ensure that the pre-perm product has been evenly distributed. It should not be rinsed from the hair so the perm should be carried out immediately after the application. If the hair is particularly tangled after shampooing, and you need to cut the hair before it is wound on curlers, apply the pre-perm product to the hair before you cut, as it will make the task easier to perform. If the hair feels too dry before you perm, simply dampen your hair with a water spray. There is no need to apply more pre-perm product to replace the lost moisture.

With Afro hair, the hair is not usually shampooed before a relaxer or curly perm. Special pre-perm treatments called protective polymers have been produced. These are usually in a cream or liquid form and are massaged into porous areas when the hair is dry. The relaxing treatment is then carried out without rinsing the pre-perm product from the hair. You should not use normal conditioners in case they create a barrier which cannot be penetrated.

2.5 Elasticity test

What is an elasticity test?

An elasticity test is a method of assessing the degree of damage to the internal hair structure, i.e. to the cortex.

What does 'elasticity' mean?

Elasticity is the ability of hair to be stretched and then return to its original length when the stretching force is removed.

How elastic is the hair?

A hair in good condition can stretch up to one third of its own length and then return to its original length. The extension of hair is opposed by both the hydrogen bonds (which are comparatively weak) and the disulphide bonds (which are strong) (see [1.2]). The cuticle scales play no part in elasticity and simply slip over each other as the hair is stretched.

If dry hair is extended more than a third of its length it will reach its elastic limit. Beyond this the hair will not return to its original length when the stretching force is removed. As most of the hydrogen bonds are broken, the coiled structure of the hair collapses and the hair snaps.

As can be seen from Fig. 2.3, wet hair can stretch twice as much as dry hair without being damaged. This is because the amount of moisture present in the cortex allows water to become bound to the hydrogen bonds, allowing them to extend further so that they give less resistance to stretching. Hair which has been dampened with perm lotion over-stretches easily because hydrogen bonds are broken by the alkaline lotion. Although it will now have the high elastic limit of 70 per cent the hair structure has been damaged.

Condition of hair	Elasticity
Dry, normal hair	20–30%
Wet, normal hair	50–60%
Hair, dampened with cold wave lotion	70% (hair damaged)

Fig. 2.3   Elasticity of hair.

Once hair has reached its elastic limit it has been permanently damaged and cannot return to its original length. The tensile strength will also have been reduced. (This is the weight that would have to be applied to an individual hair to stretch it to breaking point.) Tension used during cold wave winding can easily cause damage because of the increased elasticity of the hair. This is why tension is avoided during winding.

Because of its elastic nature, hair in good condition can withstand relatively great forces – for example, hair is stronger than copper wire of the same diameter.

What makes hair lose its elasticity?

Poor elasticity is due to the cortex of the hair being damaged. It is mostly caused by chemical processing (perming, relaxing, bleaching or tinting) which attacks the disulphide bonds of the cortex. The reduced number of bonds means that the hair stretches more easily but cannot return to its original length. Severe physical abuse such as the use of excessive heat can also cause the hair to lose its elasticity. Little damage is caused by combing, brushing and winding.

How do I test the elasticity of hair?

Take a single strand of hair and hold firmly at each end with the thumb and forefinger. Pull gently between the fingers and see how much the hair stretches and springs back. As you will be doing this test (see Fig. 2.4) with dry hair, you will not see much stretching if the hair is in good condition. However, if the hair does stretch, or even snaps, it has a weak cortex. Just like an old elastic band, damaged hair will break when stretched.

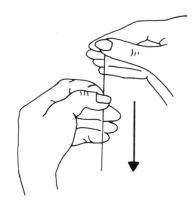

Fig. 2.4   Elasticity test.

Why should you test for elasticity?

As has been said above, elasticity is a reflection of the condition of the cortex. As perming and relaxing will both affect the bonds of the cortex it is important to know whether or not the bonds are already damaged. If too many bonds are already damaged, the resulting chemical treatment will make the hair structure weaker still, making good perm results impossible as the hair will not have the strength to hold the curl. Relaxed hair will often be extremely dry and will snap easily.

Can internal damage be repaired?

It is impossible to repair permanently the chemical bonds in the cortex once they are damaged. Conditioning treatments will help to give the hair more strength and provide free amino acids to help the cortex retain moisture. Products called restructurants are available which help repair damaged bonds. However, this is a temporary measure and the product is usually applied after the hair is shampooed.

2.6   Pre-perm test

This is a precautionary test carried out before perming hair to establish the amount of previous perm still in the hair and whether or not it is safe to proceed with another perm. (Perming over previously permed hair can be damaging and produce poor results.) For European clients, the hair needs to be shampooed and towel dried to see the amount of perm remaining in the hair. For Afro clients, the hair is not shampooed. Instead, a small amount of pre-perm lotion should be massaged into the ends of the hair which will release the curl to show how much perm there is remaining in the hair and also the demarcation line between the regrowth and the previously permed hair. If the hairdresser is unsure whether to proceed with the perm or not, a test curl should be carried out (see [2.7]).

2.7   Test curl

What is a test curl?

A test curl is a precautionary method of assessing the result of a perm by processing and neutralising one to three meshes of hair wound on curlers. By assessing the results of the wound meshes, the hairdresser can establish the following:

- the most suitable curler diameter to achieve the desired curl pattern;
- the appropriate strength and type of perming product;
- the processing time;
- whether the hair can take a perm.

When should the test curl be carried out?

Some salons always carry out a test curl before proceeding with the complete wind to ensure satisfactory results. A few manufacturers recommend that a test curl is done before using their products, so always check the instructions for the product you intend to use. Most often, hairdressers carry out a test curl if they suspect that the hair may not respond well to perm. In such cases, the hair may already be chemically processed (bleached, tinted or old perm), indicating that further chemical treatment may result in severe damage.

Sometimes the hair may have highlights. The client may be taking medication, which might interfere with the perming process. Pregnant women often find that perm results are unsatisfactory because of changes in their hair structure (due to hormones and uptake of amino acids from diet into the hair structure).

What do I need to take a test curl?

perm product(s) and matching neutraliser(s)
curlers of different diameters
end papers
gloves
cotton wool strips
applicator bottle(s) for perm products
bowl(s) and sponge(s) for neutraliser(s)
tail comb
pre-perm treatment (if hair has uneven porosity)
plastic cap
record card

How do I carry out a test curl?

- Prepare hair for perm as directed by product manufacturers.
- Apply pre-perm treatment if necessary.
- Make a centre parting from forehead to crown so that the test curl can be positioned at the crown.
- Wind one to three curlers at the crown and damp with the perming product (see Fig. 2.5).
- Position a damp cotton wool strip around the wound curlers and cover the head with the plastic cap.
- Check your watch, and then check processing every 3–5 minutes. Remember that if the hair is porous it will take up more lotion and therefore process more quickly. Also, the higher the salon temperature, the quicker the hair will process.

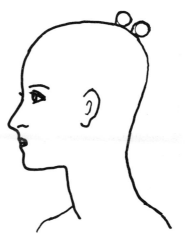

Fig. 2.5 Position of curlers at crown of head.

- When processing is complete, rinse the curlers thoroughly with warm water. Remove excess moisture from the curlers by blotting with a towel or cotton wool. (Excess moisture left in the hair will dilute the neutraliser.)
- Apply the neutraliser as recommended by the manufacturer and leave to process according to instructions.
- Rinse neutraliser from the hair and apply a conditioner.
- Check the test curl result(s) and record on the record card.
- The test curl is checked in the same way as shown in Fig. 2.6 (see later).

How do I assess the result of the test curl?

By examining the hair that has been tested you will be able to determine how well the hair has responded to chemical processing. This assessment is carried out by answering the following questions:

Curl pattern: has the hair taken on the anticipated degree of movement?

If the result is *too weak*, the cause could be related to the following faults:

- The curler used was too big.
- The processing time was too short.
- there was a barrier on the hair so perm lotion did not penetrate properly.
- Insufficient tension was used when winding.
- The perm lotion was too weak for the hair type.
- Neutralising was not carried out properly.

If the result is *too tight*, this is caused by using a curler which is too small.

If the hair is *straight* and *frizzy* it is because the hair is overprocessed. This is caused by using too strong a lotion for the hair type or allowing the hair to process for too long. This is often seen on bleached hair because the perming product penetrates through the porous cuticle into the cortex so quickly.

Elasticity: has the elasticity of the hair been weakened by the perming process?

If the hair took longer to process than anticipated (according to your initial analysis of the hair and the type of product being used), you may need to done to the cortex.

Processing: how long did the processing take?

If the hair took longer to process than anticipated (according to your initial analysis of the hair and the type of product being used), you may need to use a stronger product to achieve the desired result more quickly.

If the processing occurred very quickly, consider using a weaker product or apply a pre-perm treatment (if you didn't when you carried out the test curl) to act as a buffer, slowing down the chemical reaction. The warmer the salon is when perming, the quicker the hair processes. If you believe that the hair processed more quickly because of the heat in the salon, process the perm without using the plastic cap (the cap helps trap heat coming from the scalp and accelerates processing).

End papers: did the end papers (used to prevent buckled ends) change in colour?

Sometimes the end papers will show stains of hair colour which are lost from artificially coloured hair during the perming process. However, the end papers may turn pink or purple due to deposits of chemicals from previous treatments such as henna or metallic hair colouring. If this is the case, check the test curl for possible damage and curl pattern. If there is damage, perming may not be possible.

If the test curl is satisfactory, what next?

When the result of a test curl is satisfactory, or you have established what changes need to be made in the light of the test, you may continue with your perm. You will not need to re-perm the meshes of hair that were treated by the test curl. Section the test area neatly and wrap in cling film to protect the hair from further chemical treatment. The rest of the hair may be permed using your usual technique.

If the test curl is unsatisfactory, what next?

When the test curl result is unsatisfactory and you have established that changes to the product strength or size of curler will make no significant improvement, you should not perm the rest of the hair. The reasons for unsatisfactory test curl results will be related to changes in the internal structure of the hair. This could be due to previous chemical processing which has altered the disulphide bonds (as in bleaching or relaxing hair). Henna also can combine with disulphide bonds, making them unavailable for the perming process. The hair could also have been damaged physically by the excessive use of heat.

If you were to go ahead with the perm, the result would be no different than the disappointing test curl and your client would be dissatisfied. Instead, explain to your client why a perm should not be carried out and suggest an alternative such as a restyle which does not rely on the support of a curl. A client will value your professionalism once she understands the reasons for not carrying out the perm. If a client is adamant that she wants her hair permed let her have it ruined at another salon!

Once a test curl has been done a small area at the crown may be curly while the rest is straight. Suggest a conditioning treatment and stretch out the curl when it is set or blow-dried. It is not advisable to relax the curl chemically as this would damage the hair.

You could also carry out a similar procedure for relaxing hair if you are unsure what product to use or how long to process. It avoids the possibility of disastrous results affecting the whole head.

2.8 Curl test

This is a test which is carried out *during* the development of a perm to monitor the progress of the curl formation. In other words, it is a way of checking the curl development to see if the hair is sufficiently processed. A curl test should be carried out at regular 3–5 minute intervals during the development time unless the product manufacturer states otherwise. A curl test is done by gently unwinding a few rods (on different parts of the head) a couple of turns only and then nudging the hair forward towards the scalp. This gentle nudging action allows the hairdresser to see if the hair is taking on the shape of the curler it had been wound around. The hairdresser should be looking for an 'S' movement in the partially unwound mesh of hair which corresponds to the size of curler which is being used. Therefore a tight 'S' shape would be looked for if a small diameter rod was used whereas a looser 'S' shape would be expected if the hair had been wound on a larger diameter rod. When the hairdresser is satisfied that the hair has a satisfactory 'S' shape the wound hair is ready to be rinsed at the backwash in preparation to be neutralised.

To monitor curl development you will need to take a curl test on several areas of the head at regular intervals during the processing of a perm. Gently unwind the curler without putting any tension on the hair.

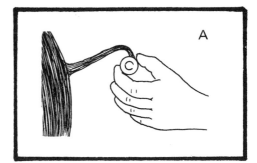

You can see from the diagram that the curler is carefully unwound without pulling or stretching the hair.

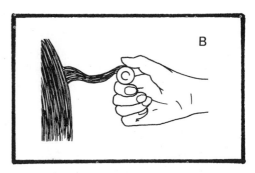

Fig. 2.6 Checking curl development.

The curler is gently nudged forward to the scalp to see if the hair has taken on the shape of the curler. The stylist is looking for an 'S' shape the same size as the curler.

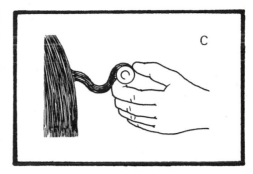

This example shows that the hair is sufficiently processed because the mesh has taken on the same shape as the curler on which it was wrapped. The 'S' shape will be equivalent to the diameter of the curler. When monitoring curl development for an acid wave, there is a slight difference in what the stylist needs to look for. For acid waves, the unwound hair being given the curl test will take on the 'S' shape and separate into strands like spaghetti.

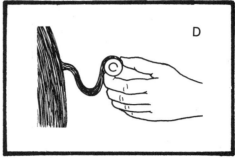

Fig. 2.6   Checking curl development (*cont*).

2.9   *Protection for the hairdresser*

Perming, relaxing and neutralising products will all stain and damage the fabric of clothing. The client's clothes will be protected by a gown, towels and perhaps a plastic cape, but what about your own clothing?

Many hairdressers wear an overall when working in the salon but it is becoming increasingly popular for hairdressers to wear their own clothes when working. Perhaps this is because it creates a more fashionable salon image. Some salons promote the wearing of uniforms or colour co-ordinated separates for the staff, but these provide very little protection when working with chemicals that stain. For this reason, plastic aprons are often worn to protect the hairdresser's clothes or salon uniform. Many manufacturers make aprons to advertise their hairdressing products, which occasionally come free with large product orders. For a small outlay, such aprons save a lot of expense incurred in replacing ruined clothes. Larger salon organisations sometimes design their own logo to be printed on aprons, which is an ingenious form of salon promotion.

When working with perming or relaxing products, your hands should be protected by gloves as the pH of these chemicals is usually high and harmful to the skin. Using such products without wearing gloves often results in reddened, dry hands which crack and are sore. Remember that the products are designed to affect hair, which is only another form of keratin, like your skin and nails. Dermatitis from chemicals is a common disorder amongst hairdressers, and when it is serious it can force the hairdresser to leave the trade. (For more information on dermatitis, see *Hygiene – A Salon Handbook*.) Special hairdressers' rubber gloves are extremely fine, allowing greater touch sensitivity than the thicker, more cumbersome, household rubber gloves. Buy gloves which are a snug fit, so that they are like a second skin. Always wash and dry your gloves when you take them off, or they will perish quickly. A light sprinkling of talcum powder inside the gloves will make them easier to put on. Plastic disposable gloves are also available, usually made of see-through polythene. They can be worn by people who are allergic to rubber. They are not as popular because they do not stretch to fit the hand snugly. This makes it more difficult to control your actions. Unlike rubber gloves they are smooth without texture and the hair is therefore more difficult to grip.

2.10 Working guidelines

1. Ask your client to remove chunky jewellery, bulky sweaters, etc. and protect the client with a gown and towels. You are liable to pay for any damage caused to your client's clothing!
2. Always read and follow manufacturers' instructions as products are designed to work and be used in a specific way. If you do not follow the manufacturer's instructions, and something does go drastically wrong, you could be sued for negligence.
3. Make sure you spend time with your client before you begin her hair. Communication between the client and hairdresser is of utmost importance as it ensures that the hairdresser is aware of the client's wishes; misunderstandings can lose clients.
4. Try to keep perming reagent from coming into contact with the scalp unnecessarily; perm products can irritate the skin. Relaxers should never come into contact with the skin as they can burn it. Protect the scalp with a barrier cream.
5. If a product accidentally enters the eye, flood it with water immediately to dilute and remove the chemical. Seek medical help if irritation continues. Using a backwash will help to prevent chemicals from entering the eye. (This is essential when using a relaxer.)
6. Carry out appropriate tests before perming or relaxing – don't take unnecessary risks.
7. Wear rubber gloves when perming or relaxing – your hands are your livelihood. Do this even when taking a test curl.
8. Keep record cards up to date – don't imagine that you'll remember.

9. Products can irritate the lungs, so avoid inhaling fumes.
10. Ensure that you fully inform your client of any aftercare treatments and products that will help maintain her hair's condition and style (see *Cutting and Styling – A Salon Handbook*).
11. Do not mix perms and neutralisers from different product ranges – they may not work properly under these conditions.

2.11 Recording client information

Why should records be kept?

It is essential to keep a record of any perming or relaxing treatments carried out in the salon. There are a number of reasons:

- You will not remember what products were used, how, and when they were used.
- When you next see the client, you can check on product performance and suitability of techniques employed.
- If you are ill, no guess-work would be necessary for the colleague attending to your client.
- The clients will be aware that they are being treated in a professional manner.
- If a court case should result from damage to a client's hair or scalp, good client records provide proof of professionalism.

What information should be recorded?

It is important that all of this information is recorded in neat handwriting so that it can easily be read if you are away.

Client's name	Include surname, forename (initials), their title (i.e. Mr, Mrs, Miss, Dr etc.)
Address	You will be able to check the address with your client to ensure you have the correct card.
Telephone number	If you have the client's home and daytime numbers you can get in contact should the stylist be ill to offer another stylist or an alternative appointment.
Date of appointment	This enables you to see when the

	client visited the salon last for chemical treatment.
Stylist	This tells the salon who the client's stylist is.
Scalp	Scalp condition should be recorded (e.g. sensitive, dry, oily, psoriasis, cyst, etc.).
Condition/quality of hair	Gives details of hair (e.g. porous, resistant, damaged, etc.).
Treatment and technique	Perm or relaxer, winding technique, method of application.
Products	Strength and type of product used; pre-perm treatment needed?
Processing	Whether additional heat was used; length of processing time.
Result	The end result should be recorded so that unsatisfactory results are not repeated.
Retail	List products that have been purchased so that you can check their success and sell more from the same range *or* recommend other products.
* Special information	Conversation topics, interests, etc.

* You can increase the quality of the service that you offer by making a note of some personal details of each client. These might include notes on whether the client takes tea or coffee, takes milk or sugar, might require an ashtray or magazine, likes to be called by their forename or surname, etc. You might also note details about their work, children, holidays, where they live, whether they play sports, etc. This means that clients will develop a feeling of belonging to your salon, and they will marvel at your amazing memory!

You can also use the recorded information to help sell aftercare products. If you record the date of selling the client a conditioner, you can then say: 'Would you like another bottle of that conditioner you bought two months ago, Mrs Smith, as your hair has looked much better since you used it?'. Although you are selling you are also taking an interest in how clients look after their hair.

How can this information be recorded and stored?

Information can be recorded in two ways:

(a)   writing the information on a record card (see Fig. 2.7).
(b)   entering the data into a microcomputer.

PERM AND RELAXER RECORD CARD							
Name: Address: Post Code Telephone Number Daytime: Evening:		(Ms/Miss/Mrs/Mr)		SPECIAL INFORMATION			
DATE	STYLIST	SCALP	HAIR	TECHNIQUE	PRODUCTS	DEVELOPMENT	COMMENTS/RESULT

Fig. 2.7   Record card.

Record cards are generally stored in a filing box or cabinet. Salons file the cards alphabetically in the order of the clients' surnames. They can be retrieved easily and quickly by anyone, as long as they are refiled after use. The system is also inexpensive.

A microcomputer can store a great deal of information, providing you have the correct machine and software for the number of clients involved. The salon staff must be trained in order to be able to retrieve information (either on a screen or as a printout) and also to be able to enter new information. Microcomputer technology is becoming much cheaper year by year so always bear in mind the possibility of using microcomputers to do this task.

When should perming or relaxing information be recorded?

After every client! Don't leave it to the end of the day or you may forget important details such as chemical strengths or development times. The results of precautionary tests (test curl, incompatibility test, etc.) should also be recorded.

2.12   Questions

1   Why should you carry out precautionary tests on your client before chemical treatments?
2   Why should the scalp be examined?
3   What should you do if you find an infectious condition on the scalp?
4   Is it safe to perm or relax the hair if the scalp is cut?
5   Can you perm the hair of a client who has psoriasis?
6   How should the scalp be examined?
7   How could you tell if hair has been chemically treated?
8   Describe an incompatibility test.
9   Why would you carry out such a test?
10   What is a porosity test?
11   Why is it important to determine porosity?
12   What can be done to porous hair so that it can be chemically treated?
13   What is an elasticity test and how is it carried out?
14   What type of hair is most elastic?
15   What is tensile strength and how is it related to elasticity?
16   What is a pre-perm test and when would you use it?
17   What is a test curl?
18   How would you carry out a test curl?
19   What questions should you ask yourself to assess the results of a test curl?
20   What could be the reason for end papers becoming coloured during a test curl?
21   What is a curl test and why is it important to take it at regular intervals?
22   How would you protect both your own and the client's clothing?
23   How would you protect your hands?
24   What working guidelines should be observed?
25   Why should client records be kept?
26   When should record cards be filled in?
27   How can they be used to increase business?

3

Analysis

To ensure the best results, a thorough analysis must always precede any chemical work. You will need to ask your client plenty of questions and may find the use of aids such as pictures helpful. Carrying out a thorough analysis will take time, so make sure that this is accounted for in the appointment time you have allocated to clients for having their hair permed or relaxed.

Clients will often be nervous of having their hair permed or relaxed, because they may have experienced (or more probably, heard from friends) disasters or disappointments with previous efforts. You will therefore need to be patient and reassuring to gain their confidence. Make sure that you fully explain what you intend doing to your clients' hair, and that they are in full agreement!

This part of the book looks at the points you should consider before perming or relaxing hair, with reasons why each point is important. Keep the safety aspects of Chapter 2 (*Take Precautions!*) in mind. For a quick reference see *Perm analysis–at a glance* [3.4] and *Relaxer analysis–at a glance* [3.5].

3.1   The scalp

Under certain circumstances the use of perming and relaxing products can cause severe irritation, allergic reaction, or worsen existing scalp conditions.

(1)   *Cuts, abrasions and sores*
       The scalp must always be examined before chemical treatment for any cuts, abrasions or sores. Any break in the skin's surface which comes into contact with a chemical will be extremely painful and may

cause an allergic reaction. If you discover this type of scalp condition *do not perm or relax the client's hair* but suggest that they return to the salon for the service once the skin has healed.

(2) *Infectious conditions*

Under no circumstances should any hairdressing treatment be given if the client is suffering from any infectious condition such as impetigo, ringworm, lice, etc. For further reading see *Hygiene – A Salon Handbook*.

(3) *Cysts and warts*

Normally, cysts and warts do not restrict the use of perming or relaxing products unless they are open or weeping. In this case, treat as you would treat a cut, abrasion or sore. Otherwise, the only real problem with perming on a scalp which has a cyst or wart is the difficulty which may sometimes arise of placing the curler in the correct position on the raised area.

(4) *Dandruff or dry scalp*

The use of chemical products will make the scalp drier, thus aggravating either of these conditions. It may be best to suggest that the client has a course of treatment for the condition (if offered by the salon) or is recommended suitable home treatment.

(5) *Oily scalp*

An oily scalp does not affect the use of perming or relaxing chemicals. In fact, the activity of the sebaceous glands can sometimes be reduced because of the drying effect of the chemicals.

3.2 The hair

The quality of the hair you will be working with will affect the choice of product and technique that you use.

(1) The effect of condition

Porous hair will absorb chemicals easily because of the open cuticle, whereas resistant hair has a tightly closed cuticle which will resist the penetration of chemicals.

The oldest part of the hair (the points) will always be the most porous, because they have had a longer time to be subjected to physical and chemical abuse than the newest hair, close to the scalp.

Because chemicals affect the more porous areas of the hair more quickly than the non-porous areas, certain steps should be taken to minimise irregular processing during perming or relaxing. Special pre-perm treatments and protective polymer products are manufactured to help even out the hair's porosity. These products coat the hair shaft in a penetrable substance which regulates the cuticle by 'filling-in' the damaged areas. This enables the chemical to penetrate the cortext at a uniform rate.

To assess how porous the hair is, carry out the porosity test described in [2.4]. Also see Chapter 4 – *Preparation* [4.3].

Internal damage of the hair structure will be increased by perming or straightening. An elasticity test (see [2.5]) will give you an indication of how damaged the cortex is. If in doubt of how chemical treatment will affect the hair, carry out a test curl first (see [2.7]).

(2)   The effect of texture and density

The texture and the amount of hair on the head will affect your choice of product system and technique.

Texture can be described as the 'feel' and appearance of the hair. Hairdressers have a long list of words which describe what they feel and see, such as 'wiry', 'coarse', 'fine', 'soft', 'limp', 'straight', 'curly', 'dry', etc. The important factor to remember is that perming and relaxing will *change* the texture of the hair. An example of this would be altering the degree of curl in natural Afro hair to a smoother, straight form – or the opposite, perming straight hair to make it curly.

The term 'density' describes the amount of hair (per square centimetre) on the head. Thin hair requires milder relaxing cream formulae, and when perming, smaller curlers and sections. Thick hair requires stronger straightening cream formulae and, when perming, larger curlers and sections.

Perming fine hair gives it more body and a fuller appearance. Although the amount of hair on the head has obviously not been increased, perming will give the feel and appearance of more hair due to the change in texture.

The term 'texture' is also used to describe the condition of the hair – because we use our senses of touch and sight to assess the degree of damage the hair has withstood.

For analysis purposes, being skilful at evaluating the texture of hair before perming or relaxing is vital to the end result. This is because the manufacturers of the products can only tell us which product to use for a particular hair type. Establishing which type of hair you are working with is something only you can decide. If you are unsure what product strength to use, always be on the safe side and choose the weaker one. You can always boost its reactivity with some stronger product once you are sure the weaker one is not working effectively.

The strength of product you use is based on the hair type you are dealing with and *not* the result you wish to achieve. It is the diameter of the perm curler that determines how curly the hair will be after perming. Therefore, if a client with tinted hair wants a very tight, curly result, the product you would choose would be one for porous hair but the diameter of the curler used would need to be small.

The same principle applies if a client requiring a relaxer has porous hair with a very tight natural curl formation. The relaxer would be chosen according to the hair's porosity and *not* the result that was required.

EXAMPLES OF PERMS FOR EUROPEAN HAIR

Dulcia by L'Oreal is available in four strengths according to the type of hair on which they are to be used:

Lotion S – for strong natural resistant hair.

Lotion 1 – for normal hair.

Lotion 2 – for normal hair, easy to wave or coloured hair in good condition.

Lotion 3 – for coloured hair and mildly pre-lightened hair.

Creative Curl by Redken is a true acid perm in four formulae:

Normal – for normal to resistant hair.

Tinted – for hair coloured with tint and up to 30 volume hydrogen peroxide.

Fine/limp – for hair which is fine and lacks body, hair which needs extra curl resilience.

Bleached – for bleached, lightened or high lift tint.

Acclaim by Zotos is an acid wave and available in four formulae:

Regular – for normal, resistant, tinted and highlighted hair giving a soft curl with a lasting result.

Extra Body – for normal, resistant, tinted and highlighted hair giving a firmer and crisper result.

Ultrabond – for normal, resistant, tinted and highlighted hair.

High Lift – for hair which is bleached, high-lift tinted or has over 40% highlights.

EXAMPLES OF PERMS FOR AFRO HAIR

Care Free Curl by Soft Sheen Products Inc. is available in four strengths depending on the client's hair:

Super International Formula – for extremely tight, curly, resistant hair.

Super – for very curly and resistant hair.

Regular – for average and coarse hair.

Mild – for fine and tinted hair.

Supercurl Gel Perm by Supreme Beauty Products is available in three strengths depending on the client's hair:

Super – for strong, resistant, or coarse hair.

Regular – for normal hair.

Mild – for use on tinted hair in good condition or on fine hair.

EXAMPLES OF RELAXING SYSTEMS FOR AFRO HAIR

Both *TCB* by Alberto Culver and *Goldys* by Goldy's Haircare are available in three strengths depending on the client's hair:

Super – for strong, resistant or coarse hair.
Regular – for normal hair.
Mild – for fine or colour-treated hair.

Now look at Fig. 3.1 – Guidelines for product choice – see if you can answer the three problems.

Problem	*Afro-type hair*	*European (Caucasian) hair*
Hairdresser is unsure which product strength to use because the hair could be classified into more than one category.	Use the weaker product and then re-apply the stronger product if processing is too slow.	Wind the hair using the weaker lotion and then re-damp using the stronger lotion if processing is too slow
Client has a long regrowth from her last tint/bleach application.	Use the mildest formula and apply a protecting pre-perm product onto the hair which has been colour treated.	Wind the hair with a lotion for tinted hair making sure it is applied only to the colour-treated hair during the winding stage. Re-damp the wound rods with a stronger perm lotion (from the same product range) according to the resistance of the regrowth hair.
Client has highlighted hair, which results in two different textures of hair.	Do not perm Afro hair if it has been pre-lightened unless you carry out a test curl first to ascertain whether it is wise to do so.	Do not carry out the perm unless you have performed a test curl to ensure it is wise to proceed with the perm. If the result of the test curl suggests it is safe to proceed, wind the hair with water and post-damp with a mild lotion according to the manufacturer's instructions.

N.B. always consult the manufacturer's instructions.

Fig. 3.1 Guidelines for product choice.

(3)   Choice of curler size

The size of the perm curler you decide to use is determined by the amount
of curl that is required. The hair will take on the size of the curlers that you
use so this must be decided before processing begins.

You can see in Fig. 3.2 how the curler size affects the actual curl size.
Remember that the more times a mesh of hair is wrapped around a curler,
the tighter the curl result will be. Sometimes, when using acid perms, the
product manufacturer will recommend that you 'drop down a curler size' to
achieve the desired effect. What they mean by this is that you select your
curler size as you would if using an alkaline perm lotion, and then choose
one size smaller for acid waves. If the manufacturer claims that their acid
wave is 'true to rod size' there is no need to drop down a size to achieve
the desired degree of curl. The reason for this is that a true acid waving
solution will not swell the hair any more than water would. Tension is
therefore required when winding the perm to ensure a true to rod curl
pattern.

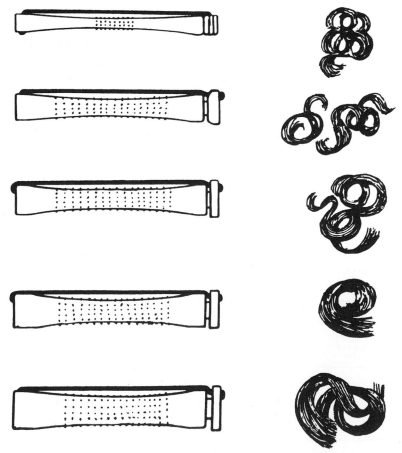

Fig. 3.2 Curler size and the effect on actual curl formation.

(4)   The effect of previous chemical treatment

The previous use of perms, relaxers, tints, colour restorers, henna and bleaches all affect the internal structure of the hair and the cuticle. You must establish the previous history of your clients by asking them questions. Keep the questions general to begin, for example: 'Have you ever tried colour on your hair before?'. If you receive a positive answer to this be more specific about what the product was and when it was used. You will have to develop an 'eye' for previous treatment in case the client does not give you all the information that you require.

Hair which has been previously bleached may have had a high proportion of its disulphide bonds destroyed. This seriously weakens the internal structure and strength of the hair. The peroxide in the bleach oxidises cystine to cysteic acid, and the disulphide bond is permanently lost. Perm lotion will enter the cortex more easily through the porous cuticle, and more perm lotion will be absorbed because there is more space between the polypeptide chains than in unbleached hair.

Hair which has been previously relaxed will also be in poor condition. It will have a damaged cuticle and cortex, as well as an altered chemical structure. This is because of the loss of disulphide bonds (cystine) caused by sodium hydroxide. The disulphide bond is turned into a single sulphur bond (lanthionine), leaving fewer sulphur bonds for perming (see the chemistry of relaxing in Chapter 6 for more information). Perming relaxed hair will give poor results or no result at all because of the change in structure of the hair. Pressed hair may also be in poor condition because of the cuticle being continually damaged by heat. If in doubt, test the hair first!

Hair which has been tinted will not only be more porous than untreated hair but will also have a tendency to lose colour. This colour loss is greatest in the rinse before neutralising, being due mainly to the perm lotion opening the cuticle.

Henna is often considered by the public as the one type of colorant that will not damage their hair. It penetrates the cortex of the hair and actually combines with some of the sulphur bonds, making them unavailable for perming. Excess henna on the cuticle can also form a partial barrier to penetration of the perm lotion.

Do not proceed with perming or relaxing until you have carried out all the necessary precautionary tests to achieve the best possible results with the minimum of damage.

3.3   The client

A perm or relaxer forms the 'foundation' of a hairstyle. Just as a hairstyle should suit the individual, the 'foundation' must be suitable for the intended finished result.

What does the client want?

A client may ask for a 'style support' or for 'more body' in her hair. Alternatively, she may request 'crisp curls' or 'tight curls'. To be sure that you and your client are both communicating on the same wavelength, you may need to use aids such as pictures, or better still, hairstyles of staff in the salon. When you ask questions use words like *what?*, *where?*, and *why?* This will mean that your client should give you relevant information, and not simply reply with 'yes' or 'no'!

Here are some examples of the types of questions that you should be asking your client to find out what they really want:

'Why do you want your hair permed/relaxed?'

- Is it to change the hairstyle?
- Will the hair need to be cut?
- What type of 'foundation' will be required?
- Is it to make her look more youthful?
- Has a friend or relative suggested it?
- Is it to maintain her present hairstyle?
- Is it to make her hair feel thicker?
- Is it to make her hair more manageable?

'When did you last have your hair permed/relaxed?'

- Is there a regrowth?
- How much has the hair grown since then?
- Is there too much perm left in the hair to have another one?
- Is she prepared to have some of the old perm cut off?

'How did you like your last perm/relaxer?'

- What did she like/dislike about it?
- Did it last as long as she anticipated?
- Did she find it easy to manage?
- Is there any damage or breakage present?

'How do you manage your hair at home?'

- Does she wash and leave her hair to dry naturally?

- Does she blow dry or set her hair?
- Does she always visit a salon and never shampoo at home?
- Does she use tongs or heated rollers, and if so, regularly?

Once you and your client have negotiated and agreed on what the intended result should be, it is your task to decide how this is best achieved – in other words, by choosing the product and techniques necessary to achieve this. From the last chapter and the previous information in this chapter, you should be able to make the correct choice of lotion.

What technique should I use?

The technique that you adopt for relaxing a head of hair will not vary that much from client to client. Admittedly, the degree of relaxing required may be different, but generally speaking, once a hairdresser is skilful in a method of applying the product (whether it be with a brush, comb or their

Desired effect	Technique
Bounce and volume at root area only	Root perm
Curl on ends of hair only	Stack perm
Bounce and volume at root, curl on lengths and ends	Twin wind
Irregular curl size giving volume and intersecting texture	Weave perm
Curl with minimal volume at roots	Pin curl perm
Ringlet or spiral curl (for longer hair only)	Tissue perming, Molton Brown permers, chopsticks, spiral rods
Zig-zag texture (for longer hair only)	Tint tube perming, Mad Mats, Rik-Raks, tongue depressors
Curl in a specific area(s) only	Partial/spot perming
Movement required to follow specific direction	Directional wind according to intended style

Fig. 3.3 Effects achieved by different winding methods. (*Note:* Hairdressers must be practised in basic winding before attempting fashion techniques. Some techniques require a lot of practice.)

hands) they will normally follow the same pattern each time. Changes in the technique would occur if certain areas only of the hair were being relaxed – for example, the fringe, the top or the back.

Choosing the right technique for perming is a more complicated decision, because so many different winding techniques are used to achieve different effects. These winding methods are more fully explained in Chapter 7. The effects achieved from the winding methods are set out in Fig. 3.3.

Hairdressers must be practised in basic winding before attempting fashion techniques. Some take practice to master, so it is often better to wind without lotion and post-damp when the winding is complete. Some manufacturers always recommend post-dampening as this enables the hairdresser to wind the perm without wearing protective gloves.

3.4   *Perm analysis - at a glance*

The analysis which precedes perming is complex and takes time. These guidelines are designed to take you through the sequence of analysis, so that important details will not be overlooked. With experience it will become second nature.

The scalp		*Notes*
Cuts, abrasions, sores	:	
Infection, infestation, disease	:	
Cysts, warts	:	
Other conditions	:	
The hair		
Condition (pre-perm treatment?)	:	
Texture	:	
Density	:	
Previous chemical treatment	:	
Curler size	:	
Perm product (e.g. strength etc.)	:	
Neutraliser	:	
Other information	:	
The client		
Reason for perm	:	
Desired effect	:	
Winding technique	:	
Other information	:	

3.5   *Relaxer analysis - at a glance*

The analysis which precedes relaxing is complex and takes time. These analysis guidelines are designed to take you through the sequence of analysis, so that important details will not be overlooked. With experience it will become second nature.

The scalp		*Notes*
Cuts, abrasions, sores	:	
Infection, infestation, disease	:	
Cysts, warts	:	
Other conditions	:	
The hair		
Condition (pre-perm product?)	:	
Texture	:	
Density	:	
Previous chemical treatment	:	
Product (e.g. strength etc.)	:	
Neutraliser	:	
Other information	:	
The client		
Reason for relaxer	:	
Desired effect	:	
Method of application	:	
Other information	:	

3.6   *Questions*

1   Why should analysis be carried out?
2   What should be said to a client who has a sore scalp?
3   What part of the hair will be the most porous?
4   How do pre-perm treatments and protective polymers work?
5   How does density of hair affect relaxing?
6   Why are perm lotions and relaxers available in different strengths?
7   How would you determine the right strength to use?
8   What determines the curler size for a particular client?
9   Why does bleached hair not take a perm properly?
10   When will tinted hair lose most colour during perming?
11   Why does relaxed hair not take a perm properly?

12 If a client uses henna, will her hair take a perm well?
13 What questions should you ask your client before perming to ensure that you know what she wants?
14 If you are attempting different winding techniques, why might it be better to post-damp the hair?
15 List the effects achieved by different winding techniques.
16 Using the 'at a glance' sections, carry out an analysis for a perm and a relaxer on someone.
17 What do manufacturers mean when they claim their perm product is 'true to rod size'?

4

Preparation

As for any practical activity, you will need to prepare for what you are about to do. In this chapter, we have divided preparation into six main headings:

- Preparing yourself
- Preparing the client
- Preparing the hair and scalp
- Sectioning the hair
- Preparing the materials
- Equipment used in perming

It is important to organise yourself so that everything you will need to carry out the perming or relaxing is neatly laid out on your trolley. Clients can easily recognise the hairdresser who is disorganised because time is wasted fetching forgotten items. Such disorganisation can undermine clients' confidence in the hairdresser at the very start of their visit to the salon.

In this section of the book we will consider the preparation necessary for successful perming or relaxing. It is assumed that you have read the previous chapter on analysis and the manufacturer's instructions for the product you are about to use.

4.1 *Preparing yourself*

Protecting your clothing

Hairdressers tend to be rather slack when it comes to preparing themselves for carrying out chemical processes such as perming or relaxing.

In many salons, fashionable uniforms or colour co-ordinated outfits are used instead of overalls. Products used in perming or relaxing will not only stain clothing but will also weaken the fibres of the fabric. For the sake of a few minutes' preparation, most of us have ruined clothing. Usually it is the cuffs and the front of the clothing that are damaged. It is evident that you should therefore wear short sleeved garments combined with a protective apron (see [2.9]).

What should I do if I get products on my clothing?

Because perming and relaxing products attack the clothing, it is important to dilute and remove the product as soon as possible. Do this by saturating the marked area with water. This is best carried out with a wad of wet cotton wool or with a water spray bottle. If done quickly, there should be little or no damage. *Remember that if it is a client's clothing, you are responsible for replacing the damaged clothing.*

Protecting your skin

As perming and relaxing products are designed to change the structure of keratin in hair, they will also affect the skin and nails (because they are also made of keratin). Many products are also caustic and can burn the skin. It is inevitable that you will get them on your hands so wear gloves to protect your skin. Some points have been made about gloves in [2.9] (types of gloves, and how to look after them). If you start wearing suitable gloves early on in your career they will feel like a second skin, and they will protect your first skin better than any barrier cream!

Protecting your vision

Nothing is more important to hairdressers than being able to see what they are doing. The salon should be adequately lit with diffused lighting which does not produce glare (fluorescent lighting fitted with diffusers is suitable). Trying to work in a dimly lit area will cause eyestrain, headaches, and make accidents more likely.

Hairdressers should have their hair tied back so that their view of the client's head is not obstructed (this will also stop the hair hanging down into products or getting caught in hair driers). The fringe of a hairstyle should be short enough so that it does not interfere with vision as well. Hair continually in the eyes can lead to eye infections and increase the risk of accidents.

If a chemical splashes into the eyes it could cause serious damage. The eye should be flooded with water immediately, to dilute the chemical and remove it. Don't wait for the eye to sting before acting!

What is the best way to remove a chemical from the eye?

As we have said, act immediately to prevent further damage from the chemical. The best way to remove a chemical in the eye is to flood the eye with water poured from a jug, or a basin handset (the hand-held showerspray). Do this over a basin and cover the unaffected eye to prevent it from being damaged. Try to use tepid water to flood the eye. Many people wrongly consider the use of small eyebaths as the ideal way of removing something from the eye. Once the chemical is removed it would form a dilute solution with the water in the eyebath, which might still damage the eye. If an eyebath is used, it must be refilled often.

We have both seen trainee hairdressers offer a client a pad of wet cotton wool to hold against the affected eye. This will dilute the chemical slightly, but it will not flush it away from the eye. Do not do this!

Try to take care that chemicals never get into the eyes, especially when using relaxers. These are sometimes so caustic that they could cause blindness. The popularity of contact lenses has made it more dangerous than ever. The chemical may react with a lens and fuse it to the eyeball. In such a case, or if pain continues after the eye has been thoroughly flooded with water, *seek immediate medical advice.*

4.2 Preparing the client

When clients visit a salon they take it for granted that the hairdresser will take all the necessary precautions to protect them.

Protecting your client's clothing

Unfortunately many hairdressers have witnessed the angry and distraught client whose clothing has been ruined by a careless colleague who has failed to ensure that the client was properly gowned. The client is within her rights to seek compensation for the spoilt garment, and may never return to the salon again.

How should a client's clothes be protected?

The gowns used to protect the client should have enough material in them to cover the client's clothing completely. The gown must be large enough to protect the larger client, so remember this if you are buying cheap gowns, which tend to be a little mean on the amount of material used. Perhaps the best type are the wrap-round ones because they are tied at the client's waist and are made in relatively long lengths. Gowns which have ties at the neck can be uncomfortable for the client and the ties can obstruct the hairdresser's work.

For chemical work, many salons also use a protective cape over the gown for added safety. Again, they should be of adequate size (think of clients' embarrassment and possible lost trade) and preferably should have a velcro strip to secure them at the nape.

A strip of cotton wool or paper tissue could be tucked around the collar of the cape to prevent any chemicals from accidentally dripping down the client's neck.

What if the client arrives at the salon wearing a bulky polo neck sweater?

Ask her to remove it! There is no way you can adequately protect a client if she is wearing such a high-necked garment. Explain the risk of damage to her clothes and ask her to remove it. In the future, she will think about what she is wearing before coming to the salon.

Ensuring client comfort

When the client has made an appointment for a perm or relaxer, she will be in the salon for a relatively long time – anything from 2 to 5 hours. It is therefore important that you make your client as comfortable as possible during this time. Offer magazines, refreshments and ashtrays at the appropriate moments.

You will have the undivided attention of the client while she is in the salon – so use it! Talk about her hair condition and her beauty routine. Give her practical advice about looking after her hair, including further services that the salon may offer. It is a sad fact in Britain that clients find out more about looking after their hair, and future fashion trends, from magazines rather than the hairdresser. It will make the salon more profitable if the client buys her shampoo, conditioner and brushes from the salon rather than the chemist or supermarket. Your clients will welcome your knowledgeable advice and interest in them.

Finally, make sure that the client is seated comfortably. Adjust the height of the chair as required. A comfortable client is less likely to move around while you are trying to work and this will make your job easier.

4.3 Preparing the hair and scalp

Never assume that all perming or relaxing products are the same and are therefore used in the same way. Manufacturers have developed products for different hair types, and there are different techniques for using them. Familiarise yourself with the products used in your salon. As there are often changes in products take advantage of the demonstrations offered by the large companies, which highlight new products and techniques. You may have to carry out some of the following procedures to prepare the hair for chemical treatment.

Shampooing the hair

This is one of the first things the hairdresser learns when working in a salon. The main purpose of shampooing is to cleanse the hair of sebum, hairspray, gel, mousse, dirt, etc. The action of shampooing removes barriers and also opens the cuticle layer, making the hair more receptive to the entry of chemicals into the cortex. Shampooing will soften some of the hydrogen bonds in the cortex of the hair, making the hair more pliable and easier to section and wind on the curlers. If the hair has uneven porosity, the more porous areas will absorb more water, which in turn will dilute the permanent waving lotion, making it act more slowly. This evens up the processing time on the hair, so that the more porous areas do not process too quickly.

In the case of a sodium hydroxide relaxer, shampooing should be omitted. The sebum on the scalp helps protect the skin from burning and helps slow down the processing of the hair. Try not to stimulate the scalp by brushing or rubbing, as it will react more to the chemical.

What type of shampoo should be used?

Unless the manufacturer states otherwise, use a clear soapless shampoo without any additives. A shampoo for dry hair might contain lanolin (sheep's sebum) which would form a barrier on the hair and restrict the entry of chemicals. Many conditioning shampoos contain silicones which will attach themselves to the damaged areas within the hair. These must be removed to ensure an even penetration of the perm lotion.

How should the hair be shampooed?

Try to avoid vigorous massage and hot water as these will stimulate the scalp and increase its blood supply. This makes the scalp more sensitive to chemicals. Use cooler water and shampoo only once, using minimal massage. If the client wants a 'good hard rub' explain that you are protecting her scalp.

As the shampoo you use will probably be a liquid type, you may find it difficult to pour into your hand before applying it to the hair. As shampoo should never be poured directly from its container onto the hair (because it will be concentrated in one place, and so might irritate the scalp) we recommend the following method of applying it. Place the palm of one hand onto the wet hair of the client, and slowly pour shampoo onto the back of this hand. The shampoo will now be evenly distributed and should not irritate the client's scalp. An alternative method is to rub the shampoo in the hands and then apply it to the dampened hair.

Should conditioner be applied after shampooing?

As most conditioners contain oils, fats or proteins that could cover the hair shaft with an impenetrable coating, they should not be used. However, manufacturers produce special pre-perm treatments that are designed to even out the porosity of porous or damaged hair before perming. These products make the cuticle smoother, thus making it easier to disentangle and comb, without the formation of an unwanted barrier on the hair shaft. You should have established the need for a pre-perm treatment in your analysis by carrying out a porosity test (see [2.4]). If the hair is particularly tangled and difficult to comb after shampooing, this indicates a porous cuticle and the need for such a treatment.

Why should the hair be towel-dried?

The hair can hold a lot of water (up to 2 fluid ounces or 60 mls on an average head) before dripping. Too much water left in the hair will cause the dilution of the lotion when it is applied. This will weaken its strength and lengthen processing time. It could also result in a relaxed curl formation. Conversely, if the hair is too dry, the product may act too quickly and the hair would overprocess. Observe manufacturers' instructions on this in case it is necessary to re-dampen the hair with a water spray if moisture is lost too quickly. Proper wetting of the hair, followed by towel drying, increases the rate of absorption of the permanent wave lotion so that it is taken up quickly and evenly. (It is far better to use a damp cloth for soaking up a spilt liquid than a dry one.)

Can anything be applied to porous ends before relaxing?

Because regrowth applications of relaxers are carried out, the middle lengths and ends of the hair shaft sometimes need to be protected in case the cream accidentally seeps past the new growth onto the older hair. A protective polymer lotion or cream can be carefully applied to the hair, avoiding the regrowth.

This product can also be used on hair being treated for the first time if the ends are porous, and so are more susceptible to overprocessing because of quicker absorption of the chemical. The protective polymer does not prevent absorption, but evens it out along the hair shaft.

Disentangling the hair

It is impossible to work with hair which is full of backcombing, tangles or hairspray. To remove these, you will need to disentangle the hair. Remember that harsh brushing will scratch the scalp so try to be gentle, or use a wide-toothed comb instead. Remember to disentangle the hair from points to roots. Any scratches made on the scalp will make it dangerous to perm or straighten, because the scalp will be irritated far more easily. Brushing the hair also stimulates the blood supply to the scalp, making it more sensitive to chemicals.

Applying protective cream

A protective cream should be applied before perming to avoid unnecessary discomfort for the client. This cream is applied around the ears and hairline as shown in Fig. 4.1. It acts as a barrier between the skin and the chemicals.

Apply the cream using your index finger, a spatula or a tint brush. Apply it by stroking *away* from the hairline. This prevents any possible barrier being applied to the hair. Use your free hand to hold the hair away from the hairline as you are working.

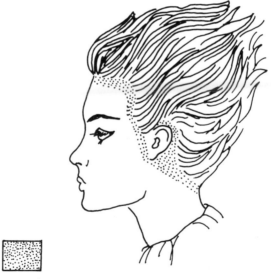

Protective cream

Fig. 4.1   Application of protective cream to the hairline.

Although barrier creams are produced by the various manufacturers, vaseline will work as effectively. Remember that in warmer weather the cream will be more 'runny' (less viscous) and may be more easily applied with a tinting brush.

When should the whole scalp be protected by the cream?

Before relaxing it is advisable to base the entire scalp with the protective cream. This means that the stylist will need to carefully section the hair and apply the cream on the entire scalp area without allowing the hair to be covered with the cream because this would create a barrier on the hair shaft.

What is the best way to 'base' the scalp?

As it is important that every centimetre of the scalp is protected by the cream before relaxing, you will need to use very small sections and work in a methodical way to ensure you have treated all of the scalp. Start by applying the cream to the entire hairline (as shown in Fig. 4.1) and then follow the same pattern as you would for applying a tint or bleach. Figure 4.2 shows how to start making half centimetre (quarter inch) partings starting at the nape, working up towards the crown and front hairline. Be thorough and careful in this area of preparation.

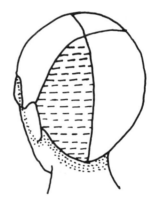

Fig. 4.2 Sections for applying protective cream to the scalp before a relaxer application.

Checking the scalp

During your analysis (see [3.1]) before any chemical treatment began, the scalp should have been checked for breaks or irritation of the skin. As the scalp would be severely irritated if any were present you should not offer the client a perm or straightening treatment under these circumstances. Ask the client to return when the scalp is healthy again.

4.4   Sectioning the hair

Whether you are perming or relaxing hair, it is important to work in a methodical and professional manner. Therefore, the hair will need sectioning before the winding or the application of the relaxer begins.

Why should the hair be sectioned for a perm?

There are a number of reasons for partitioning the hair into nine sections (the traditional method shown later in Fig. 4.9) which are wound in a uniform and specific order. Apart from making the process of winding the hair on curlers look more professional, the following is a list of reasons for sectioning.

● Aids quick winding.
● Allows the hair to be easily subdivided into meshes.
● Minimises time-wasting.
● Allows for the less receptive area of hair (for example, the nape) to be wound first, thereby giving this area a longer processing time if winding with lotion (pre-damp method).
● Can be used for most perms regardless of any peculiarities of the intended style.
● Enables the style to be varied without any great difficulty (for example, this method of sectioning may be used for some fashion winding techniques, as shown in Chapter 7).

How should the hair be partitioned into nine sections?

It is, of course, worth thinking about the relationship between the length of the perm curlers to be used and the size of the sections. A section that is too wide for the perm curler being used would result in some of the hair not being wound on the curler properly, resulting in an uneven result as shown in Fig. 4.3. Because this is such an important point, use a perm curler to help you measure the correct width, thus ensuring that all the hair will fit onto the perm curler.

The sections should be as wide as the curler.

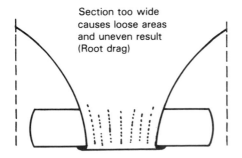
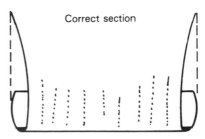

Fig. 4.3   Uneven result when winding due to taking too wide a section (reproduced courtesy of L'Oréal).

Method of sectioning for a basic perm

(1) Begin by measuring with your curler the width of the first section and make two partings that run parallel to each other along the top of the head. This section should go back as far as the crown, so will be the largest of all the sections. Secure the hair by neatly coiling and securing with a clip as shown in Fig. 4.4.

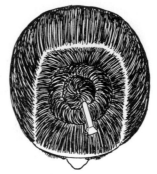

Fig. 4.4 Securing section with hair clip.

(2) To make the next sections, continue the two partings you have made down the back of the head to the nape, remembering to keep the lines parallel and the width of the curler. Divide this long section into two, horizontally, at the occipital region – i.e. the protruding bone of the skull just above the nape (see Fig. 4.5). You have now completed three of the sections.

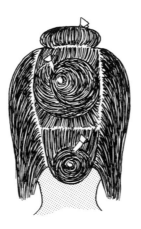

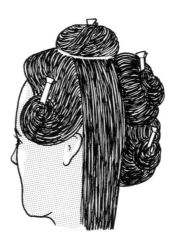

Fig. 4.5 Sections taken in occipital region.

Fig. 4.6 Parting the front hairline.

(3) Now make a vertical parting that runs from the first section you made to just behind the ear. Use your curler to help you judge the width of the section. This parting should be slightly angled so that it runs parallel to the front hairline (see Fig. 4.6). It is important to achieve the slight angle on this parting because otherwise the area behind the ear will be too wide for the length of the curler.

(4) Directly behind the front side section you will have formed another section. Divide this horizontally level with the occipital bone, making two sections, as in Fig. 4.7.

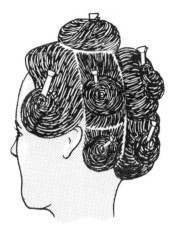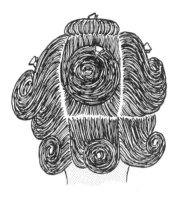

Fig. 4.7 Horizontal section at occipital region.

Fig. 4.8 The completed nine sections.

(5) Repeat this on the other side of the head, giving you nine sections as shown in Fig. 4.8.

Although the sections are not made in this order, they are wound in the order shown in Fig. 4.9. This winding pattern is followed to allow the less receptive areas of the hair to have a longer processing time.

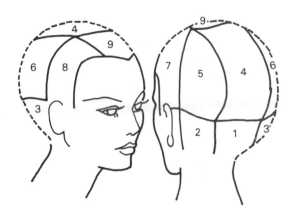

Fig. 4.9 Order of winding the nine sections (reproduced courtesy of L'Oréal).

Why should the hair be sectioned for application of a relaxer?

You will by now appreciate that different areas of the hair on the head are more porous and damaged in some parts than others. For example, if the application of a relaxer began at the front hairline (the most porous area) the hair would have processed before the more resistant, non-porous areas. The hairdresser must take this into consideration and begin the application in the less receptive areas. The most resistant area to chemical processing is the hair of the nape region. This is because the hair in this region receives less physical abuse from brushing, tonging etc., and is also more generally protected from the harmful element of sun and wind by the hair lying over it.

How should the hair be sectioned for application of a relaxer

After the application of the protective base cream to the entire scalp, the hair is partitioned into four main divisions, as shown in Figure 4.10.

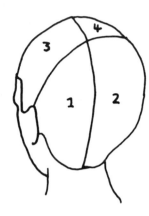

This is done by first making a parting down the centre of the head from the front hairline to the nape of the neck. A parting is then made across the top of the head from ear to ear. Sectioning clips should be used to keep the hair neatly in place.

The hair is now divided into the four main sections ready for the application to begin (see Chapter 6).

Fig. 4.10 The four main divisions for application of a straightener or relaxer.

4.5 Preparing the materials

Depending on whether you are perming or relaxing, the materials needed will be different for each process. They are set out below.

Relaxing	Perming
Protective gloves, aprons	Protective gloves, apron
Gown, cape (optional), towels	Gown, cape (optional), towels
Protective cream for basing scalp	Plain shampoo (no additives)
Protective product for porous areas of hair (optional)	Protective cream for hairline and ears
	Pre-perm treatment (optional)
Tinting brush/comb for applying relaxer to hair	Tail comb
	Wide toothed comb
Wide toothed comb	Sectioning clips
Section clips	Perm curlers
Straightener or relaxer cream	End papers
Neutraliser/neutralising shampoo	Flexible plastic strips or plastic setting pins
Conditioner	
Timer	Water spray
Record card	Timer
	Plastic cap

continued

Relaxing	Perming
	Neutraliser, with bowl and sponge
	Conditioner
	Cotton wool strips (slightly dampened)
	Perm lotion
	Record card

All of the above materials should be neatly laid out on your trolley. The trolley should have trays for storing curlers and other materials. Each tray is divided into sections so that each partition can hold a particular size of curler or item that will be needed.

Figure 4.11 shows a variety of perm curlers of different sizes. Each curler is colour-coded so that the correct size can be easily found by the hairdresser whilst winding. This code is not standard, so will not be included here – keep this in mind when referring to record cards or when buying extra curlers. The rubber strap across the top of the curler is used to secure the curler in place when it is wound.

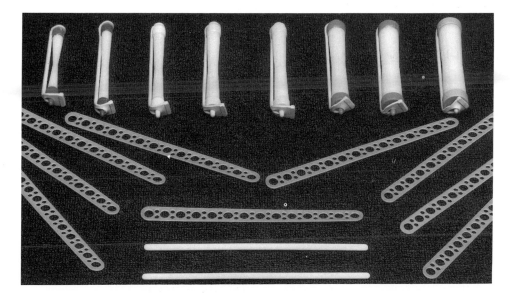

Fig. 4.11   Assortment of perm curler sizes (reproduced courtesy of Goldwell).

The plastic strips in the photograph are used to prevent band marks on the hair, which can be caused by the rubber straps which fasten the curlers. Once several curlers have been wound, the plastic strip is gently slipped under the rubber straps of the curlers, preventing 'band marks' on the hair.

Figure 4.12 shows a variety of materials needed when perming. From left to right, they are boxed perm papers, litmus testing papers, timer, neutralising sponge, water spray and, in the background, manufacturer's towels.

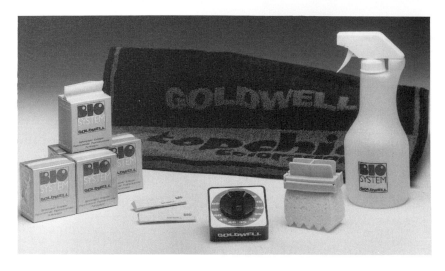

Fig. 4.12   Perming materials (reproduced courtesy of Goldwell).

Cheaper perm papers are available which are not pre-packed, ready folded in boxes. The texture of perm papers varies from being quite stiff, to being soft and crepey. Individual preference will play a large part in the choice of papers, but all perm papers must be absorbent to enable the perm lotion to penetrate uniformly into the hair. Figure 4.13 shows how end papers are used to control the ends of the hair by keeping them flat and together.

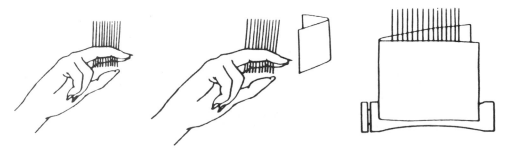

Fig. 4.13   End papers being used.

Plastic caps are used as an insulating layer between the head and the atmosphere. They trap the body heat which escapes from the head, thus shortening processing time. Some plastic perm caps are shaped so that they fit the head snugly and have an elasticated edge. If the cap does not have an elasticated edge or ties to secure it in place, gather up the excess at the nape and secure with a clip. Always make sure that every curler is covered by the cap or the processing will not be uniform. In hot weather, a plastic cap may not be necessary as processing could become too rapid. Most cold perms have been formulated to work at 20°C, which should be the average salon temperature. The hair of a client sitting in a cold draught would process much more slowly. Not all perming systems require plastic caps, and they should not be used when straightening the hair.

As the timing of a chemical process is so crucial to the end result, you cannot allow for mistakes. It is easy to forget to look at your watch when you are busy in the salon, especially when you are timing more than one process. A timer is useful in the salon, as you can set an exact time, and when this has elapsed you are warned by a bell or buzzer.

Sponges are often used to apply the neutraliser to the curlers and hair. They are made with small ridges at the base so that they fit over the curlers. A plastic handle at the top makes it easy for the stylist to manipulate.

The best method of damping hair is to use a water spray. The trigger is pulled towards the user and a spray of water is released from the nozzle. The spray can be adjusted between a fine mist or a jet of water. Change the water regularly in these sprays to prevent a build-up of green algae.

Measurement and preparation of perm lotions

Some perm lotions are packaged with the matching neutraliser in attractive individual boxes. Often, these will also contain instructions for product use, a plastic perm cap and gloves for the stylist. A large number of perm lotions are sold in one litre bottles with the matching neutraliser in separate five litre containers.

Acid perms always have two separate liquids that need to be mixed together. Lotion 'A' is the actual perm lotion and 'B' is the activator which must only be added to lotion A *immediately before* it is applied to the hair. By mixing them together too early, the strength of the perm lotion will deteriorate, resulting in a disappointing perm.

Diluting perm lotions

A few manufacturer's perm lotions need to be diluted with water to adjust their concentration for the type of hair to be permed. Always check the manufacturer's instructions to find out if dilution is necessary, and how it should be done. If dilution is necessary, the instructions usually provide a table setting out the dilution ratios for the product, which will probably look something like this:

Hair texture	Perm lotion	Water
Normal	Ready to use	—
Tinted	2 parts	1 part
Bleached/very porous	1 part	1 part or more

A dilution ratio of 1 + 1 (or 1:1) means that the required solution is made up of one part lotion and one part water, thus:

Lotion (mls)		Water (mls)		Dilution ratio
30	+	30	=	1:1
20	+	60	=	1:3
20	+	40	=	1:2
40	+	20	=	2:1

Can you see how these dilutions were worked out? Simply forget the zero on the end of each number (on the first example this leaves us 3 + 3) and see what the biggest number is that will divide into both numbers (in the case of 3 + 3, 3 is the biggest number that will divide into both numbers; it does so once for each number, giving a ratio of 1:1). In the second example, 20 + 60 becomes 2 + 6. The largest number that goes into both these numbers is 2. It divides once into 2 and three times into 6, and this gives a ratio of 1:3. Try the other two examples yourself.

Dilute the perm lotion with cold water, as the reactivity of the perm will be increased if hot water is used. Use a clean cylinder when measuring and always hold this so that the surface of the fluid being measured is level with your eyes, as shown in Fig. 4.14.

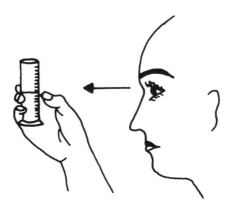

Fig. 4.14   Using a measuring cylinder.

Adding activators to perm lotions

Some perm lotions (particularly acid waves) require a special activator powder capsule or liquid to be added to them before they are used. Whether you are instructed by the manufacturer to add a powder capsule or liquid to the perm lotion, make sure you mix them well and only do this when you are ready to apply it to the hair.

Preparing the relaxer

The only preparation for a relaxer before application is to stir it. Stirring with the end of a tint brush or tail comb helps improve its consistency and makes it easier to apply.

4.6 Equipment used in perming

Some perms require the use of equipment in order to achieve the best results. This equipment is sometimes specially manufactured as part of the perm system (meaning that you can only use that manufacturer's products with the machine) whereas other perm systems may require the use of extra heat.

(1) Hood drier

A hood drier such as the one in Fig. 4.15 provides moving air that can usually be adjusted in both speed and temperature. Some perms require the use of a hood drier as well as the insulating effect of a plastic cap. The drier should be switched on before it is needed, to give it time to reach the correct temperature. A hood drier is used when recommended by the manufacturer or when a head of hair is particularly resistant to the lotion after the suggested development time has been given. If dealing with resistant hair, do not leave it unchecked for longer than three minutes in case of over-processing.

When using a true acid perm, heat is essential. The reason is that the solution, by itself, does not swell the hair and would therefore take too long to penetrate.

(2) Uniperm control unit by Clynol

Uniperm is a perming system which uses a controlled source of heat supplied by special clamps which are heated on the bars of a control unit

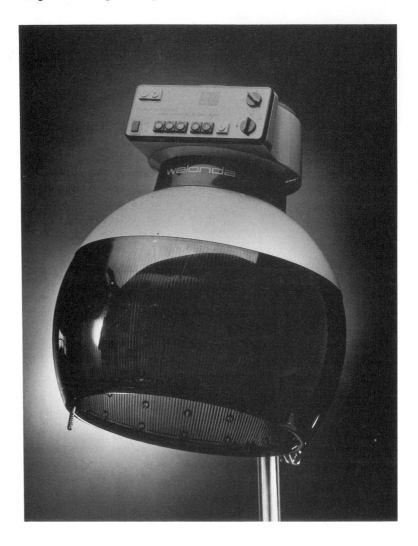

Fig. 4.15 An example of a modern hood drier. The Futura 2002 Electronic
Superstar (by Wella).

(see Fig. 5.14). The hair is wound and saturated with the correct strength of
lotion. Meanwhile, the clamps are being heated. When ready, the clamps
are transferred to the wound curlers and the hair is processed for a fixed
period of six minutes. The control unit should be switched on before
winding begins to allow the clamps to heat up to the correct temperature.
No cap or additional heat source should be used for processing.

(3) Airboy by Goldwell

With Goldwell's foam perms, a special unit is used which converts the

5

Perming (including Curly Perms for Afro Hair)

Perming is a permanent method of giving hair curl. Although it is usually performed on people with straight hair, a type of perming is also used on Afro hair to give larger curls (see Figs. 5.31–5.36). To be a good permer you should have some knowledge of all the perming systems, so that you can offer your client the one that is most suitable for her hair.

The chemistry of perming is interesting to hairdressers because they can see what changes occur in the hair, and how to minimise the damage these changes can cause. When you come to Chapter 8, which deals with the history of perming, you will see how much things have changed this century.

We need to take a look at different perming systems to understand how they vary in formulae, techniques, and the tools and equipment necessary for each. The current perming systems in use will be examined in the following order:

The chemistry behind the perm
Cold wave – *Dulcia Vitality* by L'Oréal
Foam perm – *Bio Control* by Goldwell
Acid perm – *Acclaim* by Zotos
Tepid perm – *Uniperm* by Clynol
Style support – *Demi Wave* by L'Oréal
Jetting – by L'Oréal
Curly perm – *Care Free Curl* by Soft Sheen
Points to success
Technical problems in perming

The perm systems we have chosen as examples should not be taken as an indication of excellence over other products. The ingredients in rival manufacturers' perms will be similar for any particular perm type. Personal preference will play a major part in the perms that you use yourself.

Although all perms are designed to give permanent curl to hair, you have a choice of different types of product. Some manufacturers market perms specifically for what they consider 'up-market' salons, coming complete with conditioner and aftercare hints for the client. Others aim at a mass market and you will find that some clients ask for their products by name as a result of press advertisements.

In all the examples that follow it is assumed that you would have carried out precautionary tests and a thorough analysis prior to the perm, according to the manufacturer's instructions.

5.1   The chemistry behind the perm

Cold permanent waving

The best known of the permanent waving lotions is usually referred to as a *cold wave* lotion. This is to distinguish it from the old heat perms which required very hot temperatures to work. The cold wave lotion is based on a salt called ammonium thioglycollate. This is prepared by the manufacturers mixing thioglycollic acid with ammonium hydroxide, to produce an alkaline solution of ammonium thioglycollate. The thioglycollate attacks the disulphide bonds between adjacent polypeptide chains and breaks them in two by a process known as reduction (this is simply the addition of one hydrogen atom to each of the sulphurs, half of a cystine with a hydrogen attached is known as cysteine). In this broken state, the straight hair can take on the shape of a curler. (Hairdressers often refer to the perm lotion 'softening' the hair.) When the hair has processed enough (when enough disulphide bonds have been broken) the perm lotion is rinsed from the hair to stop any further action. The second stage is to fix or harden the hair to take on its new shape from the curler. To do this the hydrogen must be removed from the individual sulphurs (in the cysteines) so that the disulphide bonds can be reformed in their new positions, making the new wave permanent.

Step-by-step to perming

The following series of diagrams will take us through the perming process in a step-by-step manner:

Figure 5.1 – this is normal hair. It contains an amino acid called *cystine* (see key). While cystine is the most predominant sulphur-containing amino acid of keratin the hair structure will remain stable.

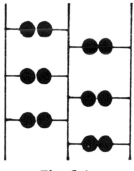

Fig. 5.1

Key to Figs 5.1–5.5

sulphur = ●   hydrogen = ○   oxygen = ◐

cystine molecule ─●●─   cysteine molecule ─●○

water molecule ⊗○

Figure 5.2 – the application of the cold wave lotion. When the perm lotion is applied to the hair the *reducing agent, ammonium thioglycollate*, adds *hydrogen* (see key). The hydrogen attacks and breaks down the disulphide bonds of the cystine molecules in the cortex of the hair.

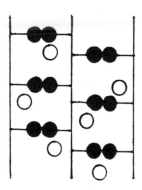

Fig. 5.2

Figure 5.3 – the hair is divided into sections and wound onto the perm curlers. This is done *evenly*, *without tension* (the hair is much more elastic when covered with perm lotion and could be easily damaged). Curler size will determine the final curl size. As the disulphide bonds are broken by reduction each cystine is reduced to form two *cysteines* (see key). The softened hair now takes on the shape of the curlers.

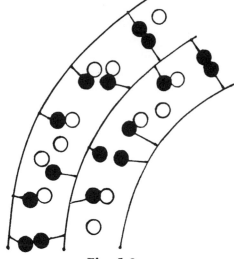

Fig. 5.3

If too many of the disulphide bonds are broken down during processing the structure of the hair would break up and the hair would be destroyed (chemicals which can destroy hair are called *depilatories* – but perm lotion is only one when used wrongly!). Most cold wave lotions break down an average 20 per cent of the disulphide bonds in hair. The diagrams therefore exaggerate this number to show how the lotion works. Once processing is complete the perm lotion is rinsed from the hair to stop further processing.

Figure 5.4 – the application of neutraliser. The purpose of applying the neutraliser is to stabilise the hair structure, so that it hardens to take on the shape of the curler permanently. (The term neutralisation is scientifically incorrect, because this, strictly, should refer to an acid and an alkali reacting to give a salt and water and a neutral pH. This is why you will often hear terms like 'normalising' or rebonding used instead.) The chemical contained in the neutraliser is an *oxidising* agent, usually

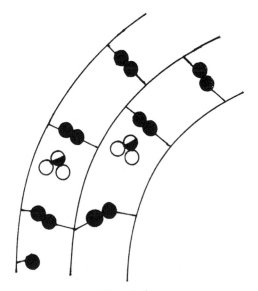

Fig. 5.4

hydrogen peroxide, which removes the hydrogens from two cysteines to form water with the oxygen given off by the neutraliser. The disulphide bonds are reformed in a new position to hold the curl in place.

Figure 5.5 – hair is normal again. You can now see that the hair has mostly cystines present again. Not all the disulphide bonds will rejoin in practice, and there will be an increase in the number of cysteines present when this happens. Some cysteines are also oxidised by the neutraliser to form cysteic acid. When this happens in excess (over-neutralisation) the structure of the hair will be seriously weakened because these sulphurs are no

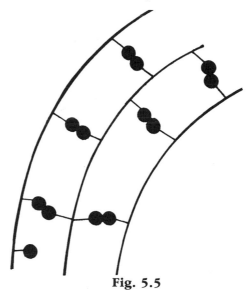

Fig. 5.5

longer available to hold the structure of the hair intact. As with all chemical processes, the hair is now more porous.

Why are there different strengths of perm lotion?

There are different strengths of perm lotion to suit different hair types, so that the hair does not process too slowly or too rapidly. The term 'strength' refers to the amount of ammonium thioglycollate and not the pH. Most cold wave lotions are designed to work at a pH of between 9.4 and 9.6. At this pH, the hair swells enough to allow easy entry of the perm lotion through the cuticle and into the cortex. If the pH were higher, the structure of the hair would break up too quickly. A perm lotion designed to work on resistant hair would have between 8 and 10 per cent ammonium thioglycollate. A lotion for normal hair would contain between 6 and 8 per cent, while a lotion for weak, porous hair, would contain between 5 and 6 per cent.

What additives are present in a cold wave lotion?

Besides the ammonium thioglycollate, or other waving chemical, the manufacturers have incorporated a number of other ingredients in their perm lotions.

Wetting agents are added to help get the lotion into the cortex. A wetting agent is a type of detergent which does not foam.

Porosity controllers are added to help control the porosity of the hair. The most recent types are plastics which combine with the cuticle of the hair, repairing damaged sections. Manufacturers guard their exact formulation closely! On very porous hair, however, a pre-perm treatment may still need to be given.

Conditioners are added to perm lotions to replace the natural oils of the hair which are lost in perming. They help to prevent the hair from drying out too quickly and are usually mineral oils or products based on lanolin.

Anti-'fly-away' agents are added to help reduce the electrostatic charges that build up during brushing out of the waves. When the hair is brushed, negative charges are removed leaving the hair positive. As each strand of hair is positive the like charges repel each other (like putting the same two poles of a magnet together), giving unmanageable fly-away hair. The anti-fly-away agents are absorbed onto the cuticle.

Thickening agents are added to some perm lotions to give a cream rather than a liquid lotion. Many hairdressers assume that they are stronger because they are thicker, but this is not so.

Perfumes are an essential part of a perm lotion. There are strong odours of ammonia which need to be masked. Older hairdressers will recall how you could smell a salon in the street if someone was having a perm!

What are the active ingredients in neutralisers

Hydrogen peroxide is the best known chemical used in neutralisers, but a number of other oxidising agents (chemicals that give off oxygen) are used, sodium bromate being the most common. Liquid neutralisers usually contain either a 6 per cent (20 volume) solution of hydrogen peroxide or a 5 per cent solution of sodium bromate. Stronger solutions of both oxidising agents are to be avoided as there is likely to be some loss of hair colour, due to bleaching (oxidation) of pigments.

Why do some neutralisers foam up?

In some neutralisers, which are usually applied with a sponge, a small amount (about 1 per cent) of soapless detergent is added to produce a foam to hold the neutraliser in place on the hair. Other neutralisers, which are usually applied with an applicator bottle, do not foam and contain a non-foaming detergent to assist the entry of the neutraliser into the hair. Some neutralisers consist of a cream which is mixed with liquid peroxide just before use.

Why is the neutraliser acid?

This is because mild organic acids (acetic, citric or tartaric) are added to give a pH of between 3.0 and 4.0. This helps to neutralise any excess alkali left from the perm lotion in the hair. Remember that the neutraliser is actually an oxidising agent, so the term neutralisation is not chemically correct for this second stage of perming.

What is 'air oxidation'?

This is when atmospheric oxygen is allowed to neutralise the hair. It is a fad which is not seen in many salons. The oxidation of the disulphide bonds by this process is extremely slow, and the client would have to return the next day to have the curlers removed (it takes several hours). This process would do nothing to neutralise the alkaline condition of the hair so should not be recommended (your client will not walk off with your curlers either!).

5.2   Cold wave - Dulcia Vitality by L'Oréal

Dulcia Vitality is classified as a cold wave because it has been formulated to work at salon temperatures without heaters being attached to the perm curlers. It contains a built-in agent to strengthen and even out the porosity of the cuticle.

There are four waving lotions available in the *Dulcia Vitality* range for different hair types:

- Lotion S – for strong, natural resistant hair (usually fine in texture)
- Lotion 1 – for normal hair
- Lotion 2 – for normal hair, easy to wave, or coloured hair in good condition
- Lotion 3 – for coloured hair and mildly pre-lightened hair

The same neutraliser can be used with all four of the lotions.

The hair can be wound, applying the lotion as you work (pre-damping) or wound when the hair is damp (after shampooing and towel drying), applying the lotion when the wind is complete (post-damping).

Note: Do not apply a pre-perm treatment or use a drier for processing when using this perm system.

Method (pre-damping, basic wind)

(1) Shampoo the hair and towel dry.

(2) Section the hair into the nine basic sections (see [4.4]). Apply barrier cream.

(3) Beginning at the top of the centre nape section, take a mesh of hair which is the same width as the curler size being used. Lay the mesh across the palm of your hand and apply the lotion, directly from the applicator bottle, to within 1 cm (half an inch) of the scalp. Comb the mesh of hair to ensure that the lotion is evenly distributed. *Do not allow the lotion to drip or settle onto the scalp.*

(4) Holding the mesh of hair at a 90° angle to the shape of the head, place the end paper over the points of the hair (this prevents buckled ends) and introduce the curler, making sure that the points are positioned at its centre. Wind the curler down towards the scalp and fasten. Make sure that the curler is sitting on its own section and that the hair is evenly spread along the length of the curler, not bunched. The rubber should be fastened so that it is not twisted or causing undue tension on the hair, as this could cause marks on the hair.

(5) Take another mesh underneath the first one and repeat the process. Continue winding until all the hair in that section is wound and then re-apply more lotion to all the curlers.

(6) Follow the same procedure for section numbers 2,3,4,5,6,7,8 and 9. When all the hair is wound, go back to the first curler that was wound and take a test curl. The degree of curl formation will help you to estimate the processing time.

(7) Slightly dampen a strip of cotton wool with water (this stops the cotton wool from absorbing the perm lotion) and place this around the entire hairline. Re-damp all the curlers with the lotion making sure that none are missed. Remove the cotton wool strip or replace with a fresh piece.

(8) Cover the head with a plastic cap for processing as follows:

Natural hair – fixed development time of 15 minutes.
Coloured or sensitive hair – check every 3–5 minutes.

When taking a test curl, always check two or three curlers from different parts of the head. If development is slow, place a towel over the plastic cap. Do not use a drier unless stated in the instructions. Coloured or sensitive hair will process more quickly than natural hair.

(9) When processing is complete, remove the plastic cap and rinse the hair for three to five minutes with warm water. Remove excess moisture from the hair by blotting with a towel and then a wad of cotton wool.

The lotion

Each *Acclaim* perm is individually packaged and comes with matching neutraliser, plastic cap and product instructions. The *Acclaim* product for highly-lifted hair also contains a pre-wrap (pre-perm) lotion. All the lotions have two parts, A and B which are mixed together immediately before they are applied to the wound curlers. Winding for Zotos acid waves should always be done with water and post-damped, i.e. the lotion is applied when the winding is completed.

Acclaim is available in four formulae:

- *Acclaim* High-Lift Formula – for high-lift tinted hair, bleached/toned hair and for hair with 40% or more highlights. This lotion also has a special pre-wrap (pre-perm) lotion which is applied before the hair is wound to smooth the cuticle and equalise porosity thus achieving uniform penetration of the perm lotion and an ever   rl result. For this lotion, it is recommended that a preliminary test   (pre-perm test) is carried out and that during curl development a   rl test is taken every minute to monitor the curl development. Processing time should not exceed 15 minutes.
- *Acclaim* Ultrabond – for normal or resistant hair, tinted hair and hair with less than 40% of highlights. This lotion achieves 'true to rod size' results and the processing time is fixed so there is no need to take regular curl tests unless the hair is particularly porous. This lotion is

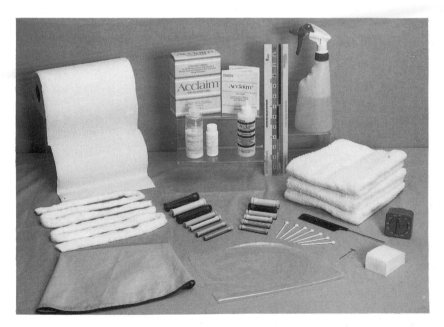

Fig. 5.14   Materials needed for a Zotos acid wave.

particularly beneficial to hair which is out of condition because the lotion contains special proteins which help to re-moisturise the hair.

● *Acclaim* Extra-Body – for fine, normal, tinted and up to 40% highlighted hair. This lotion is ideal for hair which has a history of early curl relaxation and will produce stronger, more resilient curls.

● *Acclaim* Regular – This is the lotion to use on normal, resistant, tinted and highlighted hair (up to 40%). It produces soft curls that last.

The materials which are needed for the Zotos acid wave are shown in Fig. 5.14.

Method

(1) The hair has been gently cleansed with *Duo Clean,* a pre-perm shampoo. The hair has been towel-dried and the special Zotos rod selector guide is used to determine the most suitable size of curler to achieve the optimum result. The stylist holds the rod selector guide to the scalp and holds a small section of hair against the readings on the guide as shown in Fig. 5.15.

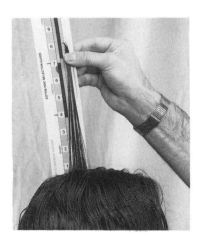

Fig. 5.15 The rod selector guide.

(2) Winding for an *Acclaim* acid wave is always carried out on hair which is damp and the perm lotion is applied after the wind is complete. Because the stylist is water winding (post-damping), he can select to begin the wind wherever he feels is most appropriate. Figure 5.16 shows that the stylist has chosen to start the wind at the crown on this particular client.

(3) Figure 5.17 shows that the winding is complete from the crown to the nape. Notice that plastic setting pins have been put through the elastics of the perm rods to prevent any marks being made on the hair.

(4) The winding then proceeds for the sides of the head by starting at the top of the head working downwards as shown in Fig. 5.18.

(5) The stylist winds the front sides and top in the direction that the hair is to be styled. You will see that the three rods at the sides are positioned so that the hair is encouraged to come forward onto the face. The hair at the top has been wound over to one side to encourage directional movement. This is shown in Fig. 5.19.

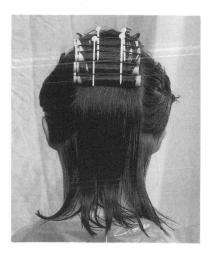

Fig. 5.16 The water wind has been started at the crown.

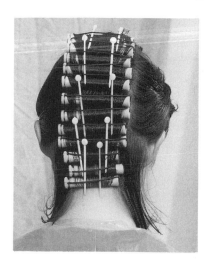

Fig. 5.17 The back centre section is complete.

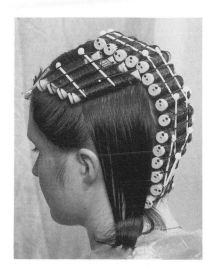

Fig. 5.18 Starting to wind the sides at the back from the top of the head.

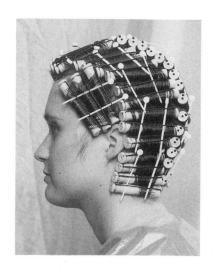

Fig. 5.19 The completed wind showing directional winding at the sides.

(6) The hair is now ready for the acid wave lotion to be applied. Slightly dampened cotton wool is placed around the entire perimeter of the rods and the lotion is prepared by mixing part A into part B. To ensure that the lotion is applied evenly and to avoid wastage, a small hole is made in the top of the applicator bottle using a pin as shown in Fig. 5.20.

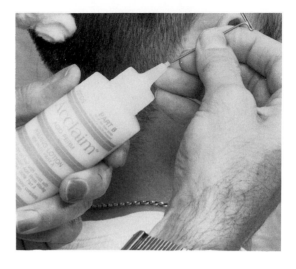

Fig. 5.20 Piercing the applicator bottle with a pin.

(7) After the lotion has been methodically applied to the wound curlers, a plastic cap is placed over them and secured using a plastic clamp to prevent heat escaping. The cotton wool strip around the perimeter of the rods is replaced with a fresh strip as soon as it becomes moist with the waving lotion. This is very important to avoid the skin around the hairline becoming irritated. Timing begins as soon as the plastic cap is put on. In this case, *Acclaim* Regular formula waving lotion is being used and because the client has normal hair the hair is left to process for 25 minutes.

(8) Once the development time of 25 minutes has elapsed, the stylist removes the plastic cap and rinses the lotion from the wound rods at the back basin. Rinsing must be done thoroughly with warm water and will take at least five minutes on short and seven minutes on long hair.

(9) After rinsing the wound rods should be blotted with a towel because excess water left in the hair prevents thorough penetration of the neutraliser and could result in a weak curl formation.

(10) The neutraliser is then applied directly from the special applicator bottle (again a pin should be used to pierce the top so that the stylist can control the application and avoid wastage). After shaking the bottle, the neutraliser is applied to the top and bottom of each rod to ensure thorough penetration. Once all the rods have been treated, the neutraliser is left to develop for five minutes.

(11) The rods are gently removed to avoid pulling or stretching the hair. The neutraliser is then worked through the hair using the palms of the hands for one minute.

(12) The hair is finally rinsed with warm water and there is no need to apply any conditioner. Figure 5.21 shows the perfect final wet result.

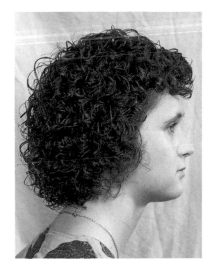

Fig. 5.21   The final wet result.

5.5   Tepid perm – Uniperm by Clynol

Tepid perming is a combination of cold and heat perming (see Figs 8.7–8.10 for an explanation of heat perming). A weak cold wave lotion and a source of mild heat are used to break down partially the cystine linkages of hair. Cold wave lotions are normally diluted by about 30 per cent, and sodium sulphite is often added to reduce this even further. As in cold waving, an oxidising neutraliser is used to reform the linkages in a new position.

The perming system

Uniperm is a heat-sensitive perming system which uses a controlled form of heat to give the hair the right amount of processing. There are three elements in the system: (i) the machine for heating clamps, (ii) the processing clamps in three sizes, and (iii) the perm lotion and neutraliser.

The hair is wound and saturated with the correct *Uniperm* lotion. Meanwhile, the clamps are heated to the correct temperature on the Uniperm machine. The clamps are then transferred to the wound, saturated curlers. The timer on the machine is then left on for six minutes, after which the clamps are removed from the curlers and the hair is rinsed. The hair is then neutralised. With *Uniperm* there can be no over- or under-processing and no test curls are required. Fewer curlers are used than in a conventional cold perm, so the winding technique is modified.

The *Uniperm* lotion is available in three different strengths. The Regular Formula is for normal hair which has not been permanently coloured. The

Extra Firm Formula is for the same normal hair type, but produces a firmer result. The Tinted Formula is for tinted hair. *Uniperm* is not recommended for highlighted or over-bleached hair.

Method

(1) Turn the heat switch to 'on' position on the *Uniperm* machine. The clamps will require 20 minutes to reach the correct temperature. If the heat is turned on before the perm is begun, the clamps will be ready for use when the hair is ready to be processed. A *Uniperm* machine is shown in Fig. 5.22.

(2) Shampoo the hair with a mild, clear, soapless shampoo. Towel dry.

(3) Select your normal curlers; the heated clamps will fit over them.

(4) Section the hair in the conventional way (i.e. into nine sections) or, if directionally winding, follow the line of the intended style.

(5) Starting in the nape section, apply the perm lotion to the hair 1.25 cms (half an inch) from the scalp. Using a tailcomb, comb from underneath with an outward motion to distribute the lotion evenly throughout the section.

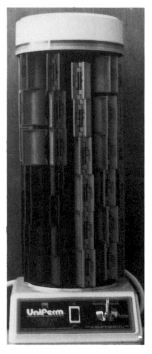

Fig. 5.22
Uniperm machine by Clynol.

(6) Begin parting the nape section, taking approximately 2.5 cms (1 inch) sub-sections or meshes. You take this depth of mesh because only 36 clamps will fit on the head.

(7) Begin winding at the nape. For each curl, comb the mesh at a 90° angle to the scalp and use an end paper for the ends. Place a curler under the ends and wind to the scalp, continually easing the mesh towards the centre of the curler, so that subsequently the clamp will cover all the hair. This is illustrated in Fig. 5.23. Be sure the curler is wound smoothly and securely, and placed directly in the centre of the parting.

(8) Wind the remaining hair in the same manner. After the nape section, wind the other sections following the basic nine section winding pattern, finishing with the front section.

(9) When winding is complete, check the clamps to see if they have reached the correct temperature. There is a heat-indicating dot on

WRONG   CORRECT

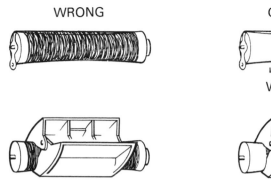

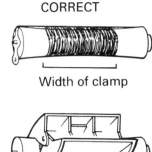

Width of clamp

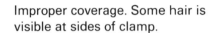

Improper coverage. Some hair is   Proper coverage. All hair is
visible at sides of clamp.   covered by clamp.

Fig. 5.23   Placement of Uniperm clamps over wound curlers.

each clamp, in the indentation next to the clamp spring. When cool this dot is red, but at the correct temperature the dot will become dark brown. Check for this colour in natural daylight or in fluorescent light; this is because lightbulbs can cause the dark brown dot to have a reddish cast, making correct reading more difficult.

(10)   Once the clamps are ready, re-damp the head with lotion. Apply the lotion to each curler, top and bottom, so it is thoroughly saturated but not dripping. Prior to placing the clamp on the curler, adjust the rubber to lie on top of the curler and away from direct contact with the heated clamp.

(11)   Place a heated clamp over each wound curler, being sure that the clamp covers the entire width of the hair mesh on the curler as in Fig. 5.23. Remember that there are three sizes of clamp to choose from.

(12)   Once all the curlers have been clamped, start the timer on the machine by turning it to the starting position. You can now turn off the machine heater without affecting the timer.

(13)   The timer will be on for six minutes when it reaches the 'processing complete' point on the dial. A bell will sound telling you that processing is complete. Remove all the clamps from the curlers.

(14)   Rinse the hair thoroughly for 3 minutes with tepid water. Towel blot to remove excess water.
       Note: if you are dealing with hair longer than 25 cms (10 inches) use the instructions in (17) and (18) for neutralising.

(15)   Pour the neutraliser into a plastic or glass bowl. Apply 85 mls of neutraliser by using a sponge, allowing the excess neutraliser to be caught in the bowl. Then dip the sponge into this excess neutraliser

and press onto each curler to force the solution through the layers of hair. Continue this process for five minutes and then remove the curlers.

(16)   Work neutraliser through the hair for one minute. Rinse thoroughly with warm water and towel dry.

If perming long hair, two further instructions apply:

(17)   Pour the neutraliser into a plastic or glass bowl. Apply 150 mls of neutraliser in the normal manner, catching the excess in a bowl. Then dip a sponge into this excess neutraliser and press onto each curl to force the solution through the layers of hair. Continue this process for five minutes. Remove the curlers.

(18)   Work neutraliser through the hair for one minute and then rinse for at least five minutes; continue rinsing until all foaming has subsided.

The perm is now complete and the hair can be styled. Soak the clamps in warm soapy water to remove the perm lotion, then rinse and dry them before returning them to the heating bars on the machine.

5.6   *Style support - Demi Wave by L'Oréal*

This is actually a cold wave lotion that is aimed at that section of people who would not normally have a perm. By calling it a 'style support' which will last several weeks, clients are convinced that they are not having a normal perm. To reinforce this to the client, special rollers have also been produced that are different from conventional perm curlers.

Demi Wave is the original style support. It is the solution for adding body to lank hair or for styles that require movement and volume. It is wound on curlers in the direction of the finished style. There is no need to section and large meshes are wound to ensure body and movement at the root. Men who might not consider a perm might have a *Demi Wave*.

Demi Wave is available in two strengths, as Lotion A (for natural hair) and Lotion B (for coloured hair). The neutraliser is known as *Demi Wave Fix*.

The rollers for *Demi Wave* come in five sizes and two lengths. They are made of plastic which allows penetration of the lotion:

- Large green
- Long mauve
- Long and short red
- Long and short yellow
- Short blue for nape hair

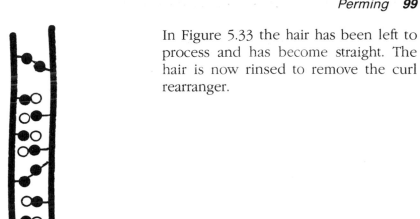

In Figure 5.33 the hair has been left to process and has become straight. The hair is now rinsed to remove the curl rearranger.

Fig. 5.33

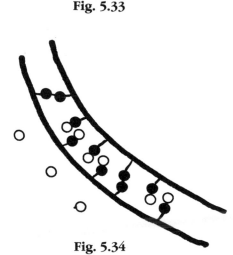

The curl booster is now applied to the hair, and this is a weaker thioglycollate solution. The hair is then wound on large curlers. The curl booster makes it easier for the hair to take on the shape of the curler, as shown in Fig. 5.34, as disulphide bonds are still being broken.

Fig. 5.34

5.8   Curly perm - Care Free Curl by Soft Sheen

When perming or 'rearranging' the curl of Afro hair, there are two main steps in the procedure. The first is the application of a chemical rearranger to straighten out the curl of the hair, known as 'softening' or 'breaking-down' the hair. The second stage occurs once the hair is smooth and straight; then it is treated with a curl booster and is wound on curlers to produce a looser curl formation. Just as in perming European hair, it is the size of the curler that will determine how curly the result will be. Neutralising is then carried out to fix the new looser curl formation. *Care Free Curl* is produced in four strengths:

- Mild – for fine and tinted hair.
- Regular – for average and coarse hair.
- Super – for very curly and resistant hair.
- Super International Formula – for extremely resistant hair.

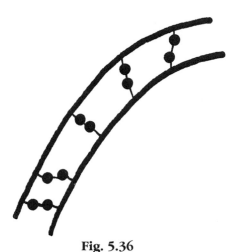

The hair now has a much looser curl formation as shown in Fig. 5.36.

Fig. 5.36

Perms carried out on Afro hair will either be on virgin hair (virgin application) or hair which has been previously permed (root retouch). Both of these methods of application will be described.

Method for virgin application

(1) Shampoo the hair only if it is coated with oils, using *Care Free Curl* Conditioning Shampoo. Use cool water and massage gently to avoid stimulating the scalp.

(2) If the hair has been weakened by previous treatment, blow drying or tonging, a polymer pre-treatment should be applied to help protect the hair and even out the porosity. This should be applied sparingly to avoid creating a barrier on the hair shaft, and the client should be put under a cool hood drier (without a plastic cap) for between 10–15 minutes.

(3) Apply protective cream around the entire hairline and ears, as previously shown in Fig. 4.1. Section hair into four main divisions as you would for a tint or relaxer. Apply the product generously with a tint brush, using 1.25 cm (half inch) sections, ensuring that all the hair is treated with the product. The hair is now left to process while covered with a plastic cap to retain body heat. Suggested rearranging times are:

17–20 minutes for tinted hair.
20–23 minutes for normal hair.
23–30 minutes for coarse hair.

If you must leave the product on the hair longer than suggested, check every 3–5 minutes. Do not overprocess.

Warning

Prolonged contact on the scalp may cause irritation. If the product is left on the scalp too long, hair breakage and scalp damage may occur.

When you are trying to determine whether the hair is sufficiently softened look for the following:

the rearranger will become thick and cloudy;
the hair will be smooth and pliable.

The objective is to get the hair completely straight at this stage of the process.

(4) Rinse the rearranger from the hair thoroughly using tepid water for at least 5 minutes. Do not shampoo or apply any other products. Gently blot excess moisture from the hair using a towel.

(5) Apply the Curl Booster directly from the bottle onto the client's hair, ensuring complete coverage. Gently comb the hair to evenly distribute the Curl Booster, using a wide toothed comb.

Special note

If the hair becomes dry during winding, reapply curl booster. Do not use water as this will slow down the chemical reaction.

---

(6) Wind the hair on perm curlers in the direction of the intended style. Remember that it is the diameter of the curler that determines the size of the curl. Use plenty of curlers (between 10–12 dozen) and keep the tension even. Do not pull or over-stretch the hair during winding, as over-stretching will damage the hair.

(7) When winding is complete, cover the head with a plastic cap and place a damp cotton wool strip around the hairline. Allow to process for 10 minutes. After this time, check processing by unwinding a curler from the back, sides and front, for one and a half turns, and check for the 'S' pattern. If the curl has not reached the desired pattern, replace the cap and check every 3 minutes.

(8) When the desired wave pattern has been achieved, rinse the hair thoroughly (without removing the curlers!) with tepid water for 5 minutes, making sure that *all* of the booster is rinsed from the hair. Blot dry each curler, first with a towel, then with a wad of cotton wool, to remove excess moisture.

(9)   Apply the neutraliser directly from the manufacturer's applicator bottle, ensuring that every curler has been saturated. Do not allow the neutraliser to enter the client's eyes or get onto the face or neck by placing a strip of damp cotton wool around the hairline. If this should become saturated, replace with fresh cotton wool as necessary. Place a plastic cap over the hair and process for 5–10 minutes. This neutraliser is based on sodium bromate rather than hydrogen peroxide; the use of peroxide would be more likely to irritate the scalp. Because it is an oxidising agent, sodium bromate can bleach natural colour and damage bonds if used too long, so it is important not to over-neutralise.

(10)   Rinse the hair thoroughly for between 3–5 minutes with tepid water until the water runs clear. *Do not shampoo.*

(11)   Remove the curlers and generously apply *Care Free Curl* keratin conditioner and leave it on for 3–5 minutes. Rinse well for 3–5 minutes with tepid water. This application of conditioner helps to minimise chemical damage and returns some of the lost free amino acids to the cortex of the hair.

(12)   The scalp and hair will have lost much of their natural oils during this chemical processing, due to the defatting nature of the chemicals used. At this stage the scalp can be 'oiled' by the use of a scalp conditioner. This lubrication prevents dryness and flaking between the roots of the hair. Lanolin is often used as an ingredient of scalp greases because of its similarity to human sebum. The hair should be sprayed with an oil-rich curl activator. This coats the hair with oil, helping to smooth down the cuticle imbrications and prevent the hair from losing moisture.

(13)   The hair can now be shaped (cut) into the desired style. An instant moisturiser is then sprayed close to the scalp and distributed over the hair by gentle massage and combing. This helps to maintain the curls and coats the hair with glycerine. Glycerine is a humectant, a hygroscopic substance that will absorb moisture from the air. This gives the hair a 'wet look' without appearing too greasy.

(14)   Finally, advise the client on a home hair-care programme. Again, this is a good way of generating extra business for your salon.

Method – retouch application

(1)   Shampoo the hair only if it is coated with oils, using *Care Free Curl* conditioning shampoo. Use cool water, and shampoo using gentle massage to avoid stimulating the scalp.

(2)   Apply a protective cream around the hairline and ears (see Fig. 4.1). Section the hair into four main divisions as you would for a tint or relaxer. Apply the curl rearranger generously with a tint brush *to the new regrowth only.*

(3) Apply a polymer pre-treatment to the remaining lengths of hair to help prevent damage to it.

(4) Allow the hair to process according to the following guide:

- Tinted hair: 17–20 minutes.
- Average hair: 20–23 minutes.
- Coarse hair: 23–30 minutes.

If the hair is extremely resistant, place the client under a warm drier with a plastic cap to accelerate the processing time. Check processing carefully as the hair may have the appearance of being straight when it is still curly.

Continue from point 4 as for virgin application.

5.9 Points to success

Dos and don'ts to keep in mind when perming are set out below. These points should be standard practice and will help you to achieve successful perms.

Dos

- Analyse the hair, scalp and the client's requirements.
- Carry out any precautionary tests that will help with your diagnosis of the hair.
- Shampoo the hair before perming, with a mild soapless shampoo that contains no additives which might coat the hair.
- Use a pre-perming lotion to even out porosity caused by wear-and-tear and previous chemical treatment.
- Section the hair carefully. (Remember that a perm is the foundation of a style so always keep the finished style in mind, and plan your winding pattern accordingly.)
- Check that you use the correct size curler for the desired result.
- Use plastic strips to avoid band marks.
- Use enough curlers. The average head of hair needs approximately seventy curlers.
- Use zig-zag sections when perming fine hair, to prevent lines in the final dressing.
- Protect your client's clothes by using a gown and towels. Use barrier cream around the hairline and ears to prevent perm lotion from irritating the skin.
- Wear protective gloves whenever you are using perming chemicals. Even the milder acid perms will still damage the hands.
- Slightly dampen the strip of cotton wool (using a water spray) that is

placed around the hairline to help prevent it from absorbing the lotion. Change the cotton wool if it becomes saturated with lotion and also when neutralising.

- Apply perm lotion carefully and evenly, not allowing it to settle on the scalp.
- Check hair at regular intervals during development if instructed to do so by the manufacturers.
- Rinse the hair thoroughly before neutralising. It takes at least five minutes if the hair is 15 cms (6 inches) long. Add another minute for every extra 2.5 cms (extra inch).
- Remove excess moisture after the perm lotion is rinsed off. Firstly blot with a towel and then with a wad of cotton wool.
- Always ensure that the neutraliser is given the correct development time and is thoroughly rinsed out in the final rinse.
- Apply a conditioner after a perm.
- Recommend a home-care programme for your client after a perm.

Don'ts

- Don't use excessive tension when winding.
- Don't twist the rubbers to make them tighter on the hair.
- Don't allow the lotion to settle on the scalp.
- Don't apply the lotion too close to the scalp.
- Don't miss any of the curlers when applying perm lotion, neutraliser, or when rinsing.
- Don't massage the scalp too hard or use a treatment shampoo before a perm.
- Don't pull the hair when you are taking out the curlers. The hair is in a soft and delicate state at this stage.
- Don't put unnecessary tension on the hair during styling and drying as this will pull out some of the newly formed curl.

5.10 Technical problems in perming

Mistakes can and do happen. You need to know the best way of coping with a problem when it arises. The problem may not have been caused by you; it may be the mistake of another hairdresser, or the client's having had a home perm.

Each problem is discussed in detail, but for a quick reference see Fig. 5.37: *Technical problems in perming – at a glance.*

Too curly

This result is caused by the curlers used being too small. Remember that the hair will take on the shape of the 'mould' (i.e. the curler) it is wrapped around. (See choice of curler size [3.2].) Remember that the curl is not made permanent until the hair is neutralised, so that it is still possible to change curlers if this stage has not been reached.

Straight frizz

If the perm product used is too strong for the type of hair, or it is allowed to process for too long on the hair, overprocessing and a straight frizz result. If too many bonds are broken, a smaller amount will be reformed. The actual slip of the keratin chains (see Figs. 5.1–5.5) will be exaggerated (like moving one side of a ladder up several rungs) because there are fewer intact disulphide bonds to hold the keratin chains in place – so much so that a frizz results. Putting too much tension on the hair when winding could also cause too much strain on the disulphide bonds holding the keratin chains in place. The displaced bonds reform in such a way as to cause the hair to take on a distorted shape, neither curl nor wave – a frizz. Such hair should be conditioned and cut to remove frizz (see *Cutting and Styling – A Salon Handbook*).

No result

The perm product must be of the correct strength, be in contact with the hair for the correct amount of time, and applied with the correct amount of heat to ensure that enough bonds are broken. Neutralising must also be carried out correctly to hold the curl. Here are some reasons for no result:

- If the lotion is too weak it will not break sufficient bonds to hold the curl.
- If processing time is too short the lotion will not be able to break the required number of bonds to hold the curl.
- If the temperature is too low, processing will be greatly reduced and insufficient bonds will be broken.
- If there is a barrier on the hair (not removed by shampooing or put on the hair by an ingredient in a shampoo, or an incorrect pre-perm conditioning treatment) the lotion will not penetrate correctly, and insufficient bonds will be broken. The hair may also have a resistant cuticle.
- Perm lotion has been used with too low a pH.

Problem	Possible causes	Possible solution
Too curly	Curlers used were too small.	If the hair is in good condition, it could be gently relaxed using perm lotion, *not* a relaxer.
Straight frizz	Either: (a) perm product was too strong; (b) hair was over-processed; (c) too much tension was used during winding.	Nourish the hair with a course of deep penetrating conditioning treatments or hair restructurants. The hair could be set on large rollers to help smooth the hair temporarily. Suggest that the client has regular haircuts.
No result	Either: (a) perm product was too weak; (b) insufficient product was applied; (c) insufficient processing; (d) curlers used were too large; (e) insufficient tension was used; (f) incorrect neutralising; (g) barrier on hair.	If the hair is in good enough condition, it could be re-permed using a mild product.
Good result when wet, poor result when dry	Either: (a) the hair has been overprocessed; (b) the hair is being stretched too much during styling.	If the hair has been overprocessed, follow the same advice as given for dealing with a straight frizz. If the problem is caused by the styling, change the method, i.e. natural dry, scrunching, etc.
Result quickly weakens	Either: (a) incorrect neutralising; (b) too much tension on hair immediately after the perm (e.g. over-stretching the hair during blow drying).	If the hair is in good enough condition, re-perm the hair using a mild product.
Breakage	Either: (a) too much tension was put on the hair; (b) the rubber bands on the rods were too tight and/or badly positioned;	A series of deep penetrating conditioning treatments or hair restructurants should be given.

	(c) the hair has been overprocessed; (d) the perm product was too strong for the hair.	
Reddening around hairline or sore scalp	Perm lotion allowed to come into contact with skin probably because of incorrect application of the lotion or failing to use a cotton wool strip and barrier cream on the hairline.	Apply a soothing cream to hairline and treat scalp with a nourishing cream. Remember that a sore scalp should be rinsed with cool water and only *minimal* massage should be used.
Pull-burn	Perm lotion allowed to enter hair follicle causing redness, swelling and discomfort. If the follicles become infected by bacteria, this will result in folliculitis.	Apply a soothing cream to affected areas. If condition is serious, advise the client visits a medical practitioner or trichologist.
Straight ends and/or fish hooks/buckled ends	Stylist has failed to wrap hair points smoothly around perm curler.	Remove affected parts by cutting.
Uneven curl formation	Either: (a) uneven application of perm lotion; (b) incorrect winding and positioning of curlers; (c) carelessly leaving pieces of hair out of the curlers; (d) barrier on hair.	If hair is in good enough condition, re-perm the affected areas making sure the other hair is securely clipped away to prevent reagent from coming into contact with it.
Discoloration of hair	Either: (a) metal tools or containers have been used which cause a reaction which discolours the hair; (b) the hair has been lightened by the perm lotion or neutralising agent.	Disguise discoloration by applying a temporary or semi-permanent colorant.

Fig. 5.37 Technical problems in perming – at a glance.

- If the curlers were removed before neutralising the curl could not be formed.
- If neutralising was not properly carried out the curl could not be fixed by reforming the bonds. (Too much water on the hair, diluting neutraliser? Or too weak a neutraliser used? Or too short a processing time for the neutraliser to reform enough bonds? Or too little neutraliser applied?) It is possible to over-neutralise by using too strong an oxidising solution or allowing the lotion to be on too long. This causes cysteine to change to cysteic acid which cannot form disulphide bonds, so the new curl will not hold.
- Neutralising may also be insufficient because too many bonds were broken by the perm lotion (see reasons for frizz above) to be adequately reformed and hold the curl.

Good result when wet, poor result when dry

This is caused by the hair being overprocessed (see frizz above) or by the hair being over-stretched during drying. Over-stretching is caused by the roller being too large for setting the hair after perming, pulling out the curl when blow drying or by brushing the curl out after drying naturally or scrunching.

Result quickly weakens

If a perm weakens or 'drops' soon after it was done, the cause is either incorrect neutralising (see 'no result' above) or the hair was subjected to too much tension immediately after the perm.

Breakage

This could be caused by excessive tension on the hair during winding, by a tight rubber causing stress on the hair, or by a badly positioned rubber holding lotion against the hair (lotion settles against the band and is concentrated in one area). (See Fig. 5.38.) The lotion may be either too strong or has been allowed to process too long, or there may have been too much heat, thus accelerating processing. There could also have been something on the hair which caused an incompatible chemical reaction such as a haircolour restorer (see [2.3]). The hair may have been too weak to process, as a result of chemical damage or a hair disorder such as monilethrix (see *Hygiene – A Salon Handbook*).

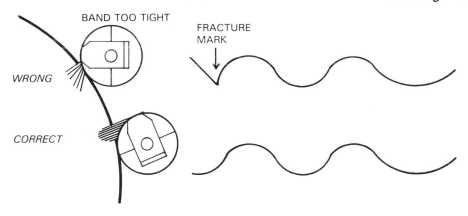

Fig. 5.38   Incorrect winding resulting in hair fracture.

Sore scalp or reddening around the hairline

A sore scalp or any redness around the hairline is caused by the perm product coming into contact with the skin. This is caused simply by the high pH of the product or by the client being allergic to an ingredient of the perm lotion. This is why you should try to keep the lotion off the client's skin. Use barrier cream around the hairline and a damp cotton wool strip to avoid dripping perm lotion. As the cotton wool will still absorb some perm lotion it should be changed as necessary.

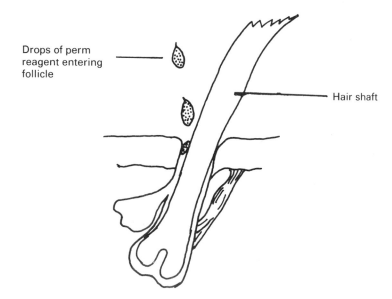

Fig. 5.39   Diagram showing perm reagent entering hair follicle causing a pull-burn.

Pull-burn

If excessive tension is used and the lotion is allowed to rest on the scalp, the perm reagent can enter the hair follicle. This causes a painful, burning sensation and will sometimes result in an infection of the hair follicle, called folliculitis. Figure 5.39 shows how a pull-burn occurs.

Straight ends or fish-hooks

The points of the hair must be smoothly and evenly wound round the curler to ensure an even curl. Bunching the points of the hair or failing to position the points in the centre of the curler when winding causes buckled or straight ends.

Uneven curl formation

When applying perm lotion to hair it is important that it is applied carefully and evenly so that it reaches all the hair to be permed and does not flood the scalp. If it is not applied to the hair evenly, some hair may end up with no perm lotion on it, resulting in no chemical change taking place. A useful tip when applying perm lotion with an applicator supplied by the manufacturer is to pierce the top with a pin rather than cut the top off with scissors because the aperture will then be small enough for you to have complete control over the application. (This also applies to applying neutraliser with an applicator.)

It is also important to correctly angle and wind the mesh of hair to be permed. Meshes should be positioned at a 90° angle to the shape of the head during winding. Winding should be even so that the hair is evenly distributed along the length of the curler to prevent uneven results (see Fig. 5.40). The width of the section should be equivalent to the diameter of

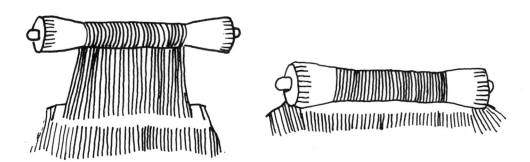

Fig. 5.40   Correct size section and angle of winding.

the curler being used, and the curler size is determined by the degree of curl which is required (see Fig. 3.2).

It must also be remembered that barriers on the hair may also cause an uneven result. For example, if too much pre-perm lotion has been put on the hair, this can sometimes create a barrier on the hair which cannot be penetrated by the perm lotion, therefore causing an uneven curl to form.

Discoloration of hair

Perm reagents react unfavourably with metal tools or containers, or metallic salts in the hair. If there is any iron in or on the hair there will be a purple discoloration when perm lotion is applied. The iron could be on the hair because hard water (with iron contamination) was used to shampoo the hair, or because an iron-based hair colour restorer had been applied (though these are usually based on other metals such as lead). The perm lotion may also react with hair that has picked up chemicals from swimming pools to produce a colour. The most likely cause would be an algicide based on a compound of copper.

Perming may also lead to loss of colour of tinted hair, because perming makes the hair more porous. The greatest loss of colour is in the rinse before neutralising. Loss of colour can be reduced by not rinsing the perm lotion out of the hair before neutralising, but you should slightly reduce the perm processing time to account for this. The acidity of the neutraliser will close the cuticle, neutralise excess alkalinity, and the oxidation of the perm will stop further breakage of bonds. Remember that if you wish to colour permed hair it will be more porous and may grab semi-permanent and temporary colours. It may grab ash tones when tinting, while reds will be more vibrant but will fade more quickly (see *Colouring – A Salon Handbook*). Acid perms are less likely to leave the hair in a porous condition.

5.11 Questions

1 What should you have done before commencing a perm?
2 What is the active ingredient of a cold wave lotion?
3 What two chemicals are mixed together by the perm lotion manufacturers to produce a cold wave lotion?
4 What is reduction?
5 Describe what happens to cystine in the first stage of perming.
6 What happens to cysteine in the second stage of perming?
7 Although hydrogen peroxide gives off oxygen, why is the second stage of perming called neutralisation?

8   What would happen to the hair if you unwound it before neutralising?
9   What is a depilatory?
10 When could perm lotion act as a depilatory?
11 What is proper chemical neutralisation?
12 Why will the hair be more porous after perming?
13 Why are there different strengths of perm lotion?
14 What is the pH of a cold wave lotion?
15 What percentage of ammonium thioglycollate do different perm lotions contain?
16 Are thick perm lotions stronger than thin ones?
17 Why are perfumes added to perm lotions?
18 What other chemical might a perm lotion neutraliser contain besides hydrogen peroxide?
19 Why is the neutraliser acidic?
20 What is air oxidation and would you recommend it?
21 What is the difference between pre-damping and post-damping?
22 Why is a perm lotion classified as a 'cold wave' lotion?
23 Why should a damp cotton wool strip be placed around the hairline?
24 How could you speed up development of a cold perm without using extra heat?
25 Why should you spray a head with water when winding?
26 Why would you take zig-zag partings?
27 What is a weave-perm?
28 How would you carry one out?
29 What benefits has an acid perm over an alkaline cold perm?
30 How is the cuticle opened if an acid perm lotion is not alkaline?
31 Before applying an acid perm how do you prepare the lotion for use?
32 What is a tepid perm?
33 Describe how you would carry out a tepid perm.
34 Why should the shampoo used before perming have no additives?
35 How would you know that Uniperm clamps were hot enough?
36 Is style support still a perm lotion?
37 How is a curly perm different from a normal perm?
38 What chemical is contained in the perm booster?
39 How will you know when the hair is sufficiently softened when performing a curly perm?
40 Why would you use a wide-toothed comb to distribute curl booster through the hair?
41 Why is it important not to over-neutralise hair?
42 Why should you use conditioners after a curly perm?
43 List eight dos and don'ts when perming.
44 Why might permed hair be too curly?
45 What are the reasons for a straight frizz?

46 Why might you not get a result when perming?

47 Why might a result be good when wet, but poor when dry?

48 Why should the perm result quickly weaken?

49 What are the reasons for breakage during perming?

50 Why might the skin around the hairline of a client become red after perming?

51 What is a pull-burn?

52 What would be the cause of straight ends or fish-hooks?

53 Why might there be straight pieces of hair after a perm?

54 What are the reasons for discoloration of hair during perming?

55 Which type of perm is least likely to leave the hair more porous?

6
Straightening/ Relaxing

Psychologically, we always want what we don't have. People with straight hair want it curly, while those with curly hair want it straight. We, the hairdressers, endeavour to meet the needs of our clients, whatever they want. One of the greatest areas for potential growth in salons is in Afro hairdressing. The main difference in hairdressing techniques between Afro and European hairdressing, is in methods of straightening hair. This chapter will look at all the different techniques of straightening that can be used in the salon today. For more detailed information, refer to *Afro Hair* by Phillip Hatton.

A tight natural curl not only limits the number of ways in which clients can have their hair styled in the salon, it also makes it more difficult to maintain the style at home. The two main methods of making tightly curled hair, especially Afro hair, straight, are as follows:

● Thermal straightening (hair pressing)
● Chemical relaxing

The two methods are different in the way they work, but will both give the desirable straightness of hair required by many clients. Straightening hair thermally is achieved physically using heat, but its effects are temporary. Using chemicals alters the hair permanently and will last until regrowth.

When clients with Afro hair come into the salon they will usually ask to have their hair relaxed or they might ask for a straightener meaning exactly the same thing – that they want to leave the salon with a style in a looser curl formation – regardless of what chemicals are used.

Product manufacturers, on the other hand, have to be very precise in the descriptions of the chemicals they use, and it is essential for hairdressers to understand the differences between the chemicals if they are to use them correctly. There are basically two sorts of chemicals that are used to alter the texture of Afro hair. The first is ammonium thioglycollate (used also in rearranging as explained in section 5.8). Thioglycollate products result in breakage of the disulphide bonds of hair which are rejoined using a second chemical. The second chemical used in straightening or relaxing products is sodium hydroxide. Sodium hydroxide breaks the disulphide bonds in the hair, but then forms totally different bonds. This happens in a one stage or one step process known as hydrolysis, which is explained in this Chapter.

You need to discuss the treatment carefully with your client to find out what the desired effect is and then decide which products are most suitable to achieve that style bearing in mind the texture of the client's hair. There are as many different textures of curly hair as there are clients. The hairdresser's skill is needed to find the particular product with the required blend and strength of chemicals to suit each client's needs. This also applies with European clients who have tightly curled hair which can be straightened with perm lotion or relaxer cream.

6.1 Thermal straightening - hair pressing

Hair pressing has been carried out in Afro-Caribbean households for most of this century. It produces good results but these last only until the hair becomes wet. Furthermore, because a great deal of heat is used to straighten the hair, continued use can cause serious damage to the hair. Also, it can lead to a form of baldness known as 'traction alopecia' if too much tension is placed on the hair during pressing (see *Hygiene – A Salon Handbook* for more information).

How does pressing straighten the hair?

Heat can be used to straighten hair by breaking down the hydrogen bonds between the polypeptide chains of keratin (check back to [1.2] if you cannot remember the chemical structure of hair). The greater the amount of heat used, the more bonds that are broken (pressing combs operate at between 1.5 and 2.5 times the temperature of boiling water). This means that the hairdresser is always trying to use the hottest comb possible, without causing too much damage to the hair. Bonds will also break more easily in hair which is already damaged (bleached, tinted or physically abused). Some tension must be placed on the hair as it drives off water and rapidly cools or the straightened hair will revert back to its natural curl immediately. During this rapid cooling the atoms of the original bonds will be too far apart to reform their old bonds, so they form new bonds (which keep the hair in its new straight form) with nearby atoms.

Hair pressing causes physical changes in the hair. The bonds are not broken by chemicals, as they would be in relaxing, chemical straightening or perming, so the change caused is temporary rather than permanent.

Water will cause the new bonds to break and the old bonds will reform, causing a reversal back to the natural curl. For this reason touch-up pressing is required when hair becomes wet.

What types of pressing are there?

There are two main types of hair pressing, soft and hard pressing:

- Soft pressing involves pressing the hair once over the entire head with a pressing comb. Soft pressing is also called single comb pressing.
- Hard pressing involves a second pressing procedure over the original soft press. As more heat and mechanical action are used it is easier to cause damage. Use caution until the right skills and confidence have been developed. Hard pressing is also called double comb pressing.

Soft and hard pressings are illustrated in Fig. 6.1.

Method for a soft press

(1)   Shampoo, rinse and towel-dry the hair. Apply pressing oil (for dry, brittle or damaged hair) or pressing cream (lanolin type for normal hair condition, sometimes called cream press) sparingly in sections over the entire head of hair. These oils and creams make it easier for the comb to move through the hair during pressing, causing less mechanical damage (they act as a lubricant and help conduct heat from the comb into the hair, making pressing quicker and more efficient).

(2)   Comb the hair and section into four quarters, clipping back three sections, leaving the back left (or right) section ready for sub-sectioning. This method of sectioning was shown earlier in Fig. 4.2.

(3)   Heat the pressing comb ready to commence pressing. Before using the comb on the hair, test the heated comb on a piece of white tissue paper before applying it to the hair. If the paper shows signs of scorching (a yellowing or browning of the paper), allow the comb to cool and retest before proceeding with pressing.

(4)   Starting at the bottom of the left (or right) back section, sub-section the hair into shorter partings and work from the nape to the crown. Clip back the hair above the sub-sections that you are working on, and complete one quarter of the head at a time. Hair which is fine and sparse can be sub-sectioned into partings larger than 3.75 cm (1½

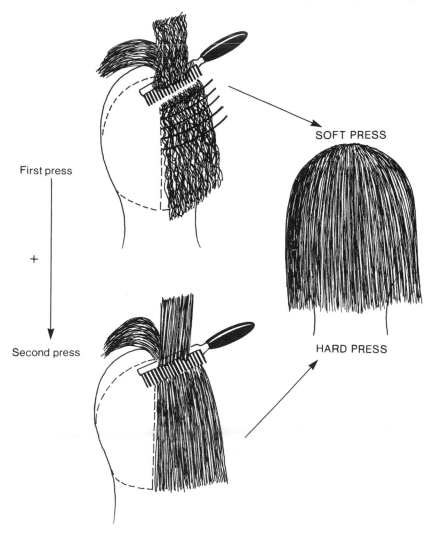

First press

+

Second press

SOFT PRESS

HARD PRESS

Fig. 6.1   The soft press is achieved by pressing the hair once, while the hard press is achieved by pressing the straightened hair a second time.

inches) while coarse hair can be sub-sectioned into smaller partings than 2.5 cm (one inch) in order to ensure complete heat penetration into the hair.

(5) Hold the ends of the hair of the sub-section between the middle and index finger of the left hand, and hold the section upward, away from the scalp. Insert the teeth of the pressing comb into the top side of the hair section close to the scalp (about one centimetre or half an inch away) holding the hair strand firmly against the back rod of the comb.

(6) Keeping a firm pressure of hair against the back rod of the pressing

comb, comb through the hair a short distance while turning the comb away from you so that the hair partly wraps itself around the comb. Maintain the pressure and draw the comb up through the entire hair strand until the hair ends pass through the teeth. This is shown in Fig. 6.2. It is the back rod of the comb that actually presses the hair. Repeat this pressing motion a second time on top of the sub-section and then reverse the comb and press the sub-section once from underneath.

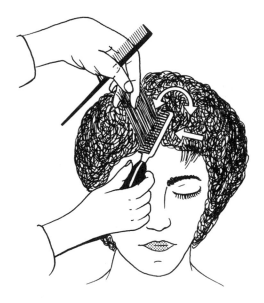

Fig. 6.2 The correct way to handle a pressing comb.

(7) Continue pressing over the quarter head section until complete, then press the other three quarter head sections until the entire head has been pressed.

Depending on the result achieved, it may be necessary to repeat pressing to get really smooth results. Coarse, wiry hair will be the most difficult for achieving good pressing results. The second pressing is achieved by repeating steps 2–7. Less pressing oil or cream is required but great care must be taken not to damage the hair.

Touch-ups may be required if parts of the hair begin to revert to their natural curl, as might occur from excessive scalp sweating.

Apply finishing/styling product to the hair near the scalp and brush it through the hair. Style and comb the hair according to the finished look the client desires. Thermal waving, curling or blow-dry styling are all popular.

6.2 Chemical hair relaxing

Chemical relaxing is a very popular service in salons dealing with Afro hair because super-curly hair can be difficult to manage and style. There are many white people, too, who prefer their hair, whether it is super-curly or slightly wavy, to be straighter.

Generally speaking, products designed for Afro hair are only used on European hair if the degree of curl formation is very tight. If the hair of a European is slightly curly or wavy and a straighter look is required, this can be achieved by using a perm lotion. Taking this into consideration, we need to look at some different methods of chemically relaxing Afro hair and tightly curly European hair.

Relaxing hair with a sodium hydroxide-based product designed for Afro-type hair has two distinct stages:

(1) The relaxer product (a thick cream) is applied to the parts of the hair to be relaxed, whether it is a virgin application or a root re-touch. The relaxer causes a chemical process called hydrolysis to take place in which disulphide bonds in the hair are broken. This has the effect of 'softening' the hair and making the curl formation relax.
(2) After the hair is sufficiently processed, the relaxer is removed by thorough rinsing. A neutralising shampoo is then used to counteract the alkalinity of the relaxer and restore the hair back to its natural pH (i.e. 4.5–5.5). In the relaxing process the neutralising shampoo does not play any part in reforming the disulphide bonds as it does in the perming process when the active chemical is ammonium thioglycollate.

What is the active ingredient of relaxers?

The main active ingredient of a relaxer is sodium hydroxide. This is a highly caustic substance, having a pH of between 10 and 14. The common name used for sodium hydroxide in the United States (where most of these products are manufactured) is lye. You may come across products which claim to contain no lye. Don't be fooled into thinking that these products are milder because if they do not contain sodium hydroxide, they will contain an equally caustic substance such as potassium or lithium hydroxide. It is interesting to note that the amount of sodium hydroxide permitted in relaxers in the United States is 10 per cent, while in the UK 4.5 is the maximum strength allowed for professional relaxer products. Beware of imitations too! Manufacturers are constantly battling with illegally made relaxer products which are finding their way to market stalls and small shops. These are usually produced in back street factories and are made to look convincingly like the real thing. Sometimes they are even packaged in the original containers to look deceptively like the real thing. However, the makers of these rogue products are only doing it to make money and are not concerned about adhering to the safety recommendations. You have been warned!

The latest products used in the United States to straighten Afro hair contain reducing agents such as sodium or ammonium bisulphite. They are milder in use than ammonium thioglycollate and can be produced with a pH of between 6.5 and 8.5. Heat is used during chemical processing. These are the equivalent of acid perms but have not gained the same widespread popularity – yet. (This is mainly because the results do not last as well as ammonium thioglycollate or sodium hydroxide relaxers.)

Method for chemically relaxing virgin Afro hair

(1)   Select the appropriate strength and type of relaxer for the client hair type. If the hair is tinted, weaker strength products should be used. If you are unsure what strength is appropriate, carry out a precautionary test. You should be sure whether you are using an ammonium thioglycollate or sodium hydroxide-based relaxer as this will affect what you do do in part (7) of this section.

(2)   Section the hair from forehead to nape, and across the top of the head from ear to ear, as shown in Fig. 4.10. Clip the hair in place (check manufacturer's instructions to see if the scalp must be based to protect it – basing is described in [4.3]). Use a protective cream around the hairline and ears to protect the skin.

(3)   Put on protective rubber gloves before starting to apply the relaxer. Start at the bottom of the right hand nape section, making narrow half centimetre (quarter inch) sub-sections, and gradually work up towards the crown. Apply the relaxer to the entire strand, starting a half to one centimetre (quarter to a half an inch) from the scalp on each sub-section. Use the back of a tailcomb or a flat tinting brush to apply the relaxer to the hair.

(4)   Repeat the procedure described until all four sections have been completed in a clockwise direction from the first section.

(5)   Let the hair process for between 5 to 15 minutes, then comb through gently with a wide-toothed comb to straighten the hair. Make sure to smooth the hair nearest the scalp. Care should be taken not to stretch the hair too much at this stage, as it is fragile and could easily be damaged. Some hairdressers use their hands instead of a comb to smooth the hair. The weight of the cream should hold the hair in place. Allow the hair to process for the time recommended by the manufacturer. Check a strand of the hair every three minutes to see if processing is complete.

(6) Once processing is complete, take the client to a backwash basin. Rinse the relaxer from the hair using warm water. Use the force of the water spray to remove the product while keeping the hair straight. Blot the hair dry with a towel.

(7) (a) *For ammonium thioglycollate-based relaxers* place a plastic container in the backwash basin. Pour neutraliser through the hair. Use the excess neutraliser which goes into the bowl to pour through the hair again. Follow manufacturer's instructions to time the neutralising. Remove any tangles before rinsing. Thoroughly rinse the neutralising solution from the hair and blot the hair dry with a towel. Condition the hair and set into desired style.

   (b) *For sodium hydroxide-based relaxers* a neutralising shampoo should be used as supplied by the manufacturer, to neutralise the alkalinity of any relaxer left on the hair. Condition and set the hair into the desired style.

Regrowth application

The procedure for a regrowth application is the same as has just been outlined above, except that the relaxer is applied only to the new hair regrowth.

In order to avoid overlapping treated hair a cream conditioner could be applied to the previously treated hair with the fingers. The previously treated hair would be very porous and could easily be overprocessed, resulting in damage and possible colour fade.

Straightening European (Caucasian) hair

Hairdressers perm hair to achieve particular styles yet they are often apprehensive when it comes to reducing the amount of curl in a head of hair. Because relaxing the hair usually entails using the same (ammonium thioglycollate) products as would be used to make straight hair curly, there is no need for concern as you are really reverse-perming. The only time a perm lotion cannot be used is when very curly hair needs to be relaxed. Liquid perm lotions would not coat the hair as well as a relaxer used for Afro hair, and could not help 'hold' the hair in its straightened position. Never attempt to straighten using a foam perm, as this is designed to be applied to hair wound on curlers. When using a perm lotion to straighten, the stylist works with a product on the hair, which is chosen according to the client's hair type and texture.

Method – straightening European hair using perm lotion

(1) Analyse the hair, scalp and the client's requirements. Shampoo and towel dry the hair. Apply a pre-perm lotion if the hair is porous.

(2)   Apply a barrier cream to the hairline and ears and then divide the hair into four main sections as in Figure 4.10.

(3)   Start by taking a 1 cm (half inch) deep mesh at the bottom of section number 1. Lay the mesh over the palm of your gloved hand and apply the perm lotion to the hair using a tint brush. Apply the lotion within 1 cm (half inch) of the scalp and comb the hair with a tail comb to make sure the lotion is evenly distributed. *Do not allow the lotion to settle on the scalp.*

(4)   Continue taking 1 cm (half inch) meshes working upwards towards the crown. When the number 1 section is completed, repeat the procedure on the other back section.

(5)   When both sections are completed, begin work on the side sections, remembering to keep the hair back from the face. Always finish your application with the front hairline as this is normally the most porous area and it will process more quickly than other areas.

(6)   When the application is complete, smooth the hair by gentle combing. It is important to use a comb with wide teeth, and not to stretch the hair with unnecessary tension during combing. Some stylists prefer to smooth the hair by using their hands at this stage. Take each mesh in turn between the hands and gently press the hair while running the joined hands from roots to tips.

(7)   Do not cover the head with a plastic cap for processing as this would disturb the hair. You will need to stay with your client during the processing stage to continue smoothing the hair. Remember to keep the hair combed back off the face to prevent dripping. As you smooth the hair it will gradually become more relaxed and will not spring back into waves or curls. When the desired degree of relaxation is achieved the hair is ready to be neutralised.

(8)   When neutralising, it is essential to use a backwash basin, as it lessens the chance of any chemicals entering the eyes (see Figure 6.3).

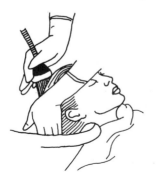

When you position the client at the backwash, carefully lay the hair into the basin with as little disturbance as possible. Rinse the hair thoroughly using warm water for at least three minutes. To remove the excess moisture from the hair, gently press a towel against the head. If the hair is long, gently press the ends of the hair between a towel.

Fig. 6.3   Using the backwash basin to rinse the client's hair. This is safer than a frontwash as there is less chance of chemicals entering the client's eyes.

(9)   Apply the neutraliser using a sponge. Make sure that the neutraliser penetrates right through the hair. Try to keep the hair in its new straight shape all the time.

(10)   As the hair is not wound on curlers, there is no need to apply the neutraliser twice. Instead, allow the hair the full development time of the neutraliser.

(11)   When the development of the neutraliser is complete, rinse the hair thoroughly and apply a conditioner.

(12)   The hair is now ready for further styling.

This straightening technique can also be used to relax gently a perm that is too tight as long as the hair is in good enough condition and has not been over-processed. As previously permed hair is already chemically processed and therefore porous, use a pre-perm lotion and proceed with caution.

Straightening hair using Mad Mats

Mad Mats are featured in Chapter 7 but are also mentioned here because they can also be used to straighten European hair by using them flat.

The hair is divided into sections and the process is usually started at the nape. Approximately 2 cm (just less than an inch) deep meshes are taken the width of the Mad Mat. The mesh is combed flat over the Mad Mat and a perm lotion is applied to the hair. The Mat is folded in half lengthways to hold the hair in the straight position. The hair is worked in this way until all the hair is wrapped. It is then processed and neutralised in the usual way, although the Mats may need to be opened slightly to ensure thorough rinsing and the penetration of the neutraliser.

6.3   General rules for relaxing

A few general rules about relaxers that contain sodium hydroxide (or other metal hydroxides) are appropriate here:

- Never relax hair if the scalp is infected or cut.
- Always wear gloves and wash the chemical off unprotected skin immediately.
- Always use a backwash. If the chemical enters the eye flood with cold water until stinging stops and seek medical advice as it is possible to blind a client.
- Read the manufacturer's instructions carefully before using the product.
- Do not shampoo the hair before applying the relaxer – the natural oils help to protect the scalp so should not be removed by shampooing. (Hair should not have been shampooed for the previous three days.)
- Apply barrier cream to the hairline and ears to protect the skin.
- Base the scalp with barrier cream because sodium hydroxide can seriously burn the scalp if it is in prolonged contact. If basing is

recommended and you have ignored it, a client will have the right to sue you for compensation. Many clients take burns for granted as a price they pay for having straight hair. They should not have to. Hairdressers often tell clients that they have dermatitis when in fact their skins are burnt. Sometimes this results in permanent scarring.

- If irritation should occur, wash the product from the hair immediately with a lot of cool water. Then use the manufacturer's neutralising shampoo, which is acid, to counteract the alkalinity. Don't assume that any discomfort will go away if you leave the chemical on a little longer – it won't! You can test the pH of your products with universal indicator paper, available from your chemist.
- Sodium hydroxide can be used to clean drains which are blocked up with hair; it simply dissolves it! It is also used to prepare skeletons for medical use by dissolving flesh off the bones. *Take care!*
- If a relaxer is sold in pots sealed with foil do not accept pots where the foil has been broken prior to purchase. The product may have gone off and you will not achieve a proper result.
- If a client has scarring on the scalp from previous straightening or relaxing, make a note on the record card. This is essential in case of clients' complaints or legal action.

Chemistry of relaxing using sodium hydroxide

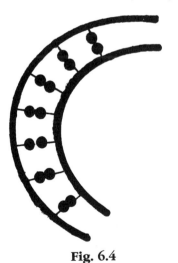

Figure 6.4 shows the natural tight curl formation of the client.

Fig. 6.4

Key to Figs 6.4–6.7

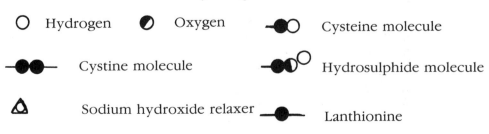

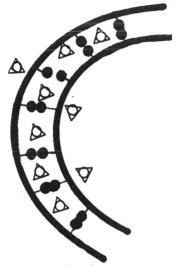

Fig. 6.5

In Fig. 6.5, the sodium hydroxide relaxer is applied to the hair. It starts to break down the disulphide bonds of cystine. The chemical process is called *hydrolysis*, and involves the chemical addition of water (not just hydrogen) to the disulphide bond.

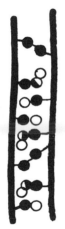

Fig. 6.6

In Fig. 6.6 the hair straightens out. The reactions involved here are extremely complex. Basically, water reacts with one of the sulphurs from the disulphide bond to form hydrosulphide while the other sulphur atom is joined by a hydrogen to give cysteine. The other half of the cystine which has lost its sulphur will begin to react with the cysteine to form a new amino acid called *lanthionine*.

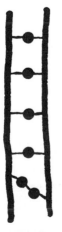

Fig. 6.7

Fig. 6.7 shows the lanthionine that has been formed. The only difference between it and cystine is that it contains only one sulphur. The hair is rinsed to remove the relaxer or the hair structure would break down. The neutralising shampoo is acidic to counteract the alkalinity of the relaxer. Unlike neutralisers used with thioglycollate, it does not reform sulphur bonds. The amino acid lysine, present in natural hair, may react to form lysinoalanine, which will also help to keep the hair straight. (N.B. neither lanthionine or lysinoalanine appear in normal hair.)

Why can't relaxed hair be permed?

One of the most frequently asked questions is: 'Why can't you perm over hair which has been relaxed?'. The answer is that the lanthionine that is formed in the hair has so few disulphide bonds left to reduce that a perm lotion cannot work successfully. This is similar to highly bleached hair, which will lose some of its disulphide bonds due to oxidation damage.

TCB Creme Hair Relaxer by Alberto Culver

This product is described as a 'no-base' relaxer because the manufacturers maintain that basing the scalp is unnecessary if the application of the relaxer is carefully done. However, you must not, *under any circumstances*, use a no-base relaxer if the client has a sensitive scalp. Also, if you are inexperienced at applying relaxers, we urge you to base the scalp as a precaution, using a barrier cream. Care should be taken not to coat the hair when basing as this will form a barrier on the hair.

This product is available in three formulae:

● Mild – for fine or colour-treated hair.
● Regular – for normal hair.
● Super – for stubborn and resistant hair.

Note: Do not use any of the above on hair which is bleached or badly damaged. The maximum processing time should not exceed eighteen minutes, including the five minutes application time.

Method – for a virgin application

(1) Prepare the client, scalp, hair and materials. *Do not shampoo the hair*.
(2) Divide the hair into four equal sections as in Fig. 4.10.
(3) Beginning at the nape of section 1, make 0.5 cm (quarter inch) partings and apply the relaxer cream using a tinting brush or your gloved fingers if you prefer. Extend the application as far down each strand as you feel there is healthy hair. Porous ends will process more quickly, so the relaxer can be applied to such areas after the initial application to the healthy areas is complete. Apply the relaxer as close to the roots as possible without it coming into contact with the scalp.
(4) Continue working upwards using narrow partings up to the crown. Repeat the application on the other back section.
(5) Apply the relaxer to the front sections, keeping the hair held away from the face. Do not apply the product to the front hairline until last, as this will process more quickly, due to the extra porosity of the hair in this area.

(6) Check the application by returning to the first section, part off a narrow mesh of hair and apply more relaxer. Follow the same pattern of application as before, making sure that no areas have been missed.

(7) Return to the first section again. Using a 'scissor-like' grip on each mesh of hair, distribute the relaxer down the entire length of the hair shaft. Repeat this in each section, making sure that all the hair is covered with the relaxer. The scissor-like grip not only spreads the product down the hair shaft but also helps to smooth the hair.

(8) Check the processing by cleaning the relaxer off a small mesh of hair and assessing the wave pattern. As a general indication for checking processing, the hair will look smooth and shiny if it is ready. Do not exceed the manufacturer's recommended processing time.

(9) Rinse the hair thoroughly at the backwash basin, making sure that all the relaxer cream is removed. Shampoo the hair twice with the special neutralising shampoo, using minimum friction from your hands. This neutralising shampoo is acidic and does not work in the same way as the neutraliser described in 7(b) on page 121 (it does not cause sulphur bonds to reform). It does, however, neutralise the alkalinity of the hair by virtue of being acidic. After the neutralising shampoo, use a rich, non-alkaline shampoo such as the TCB Super Detangling Shampoo. Figure 6.8 shows a relaxed head of Afro hair.

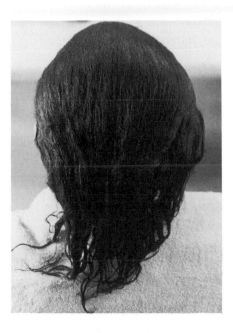

Fig. 6.8 A relaxed head of Afro hair ready for further styling.

On European hair reverse this process, so that the residue of grease is removed with a normal shampoo, and followed by the neutralising shampoo.

(10) Condition and style as normal. Suggest a home hair-care programme to your client.

Regrowth application of a relaxer

As the new curly hair grows after a relaxer, a regrowth will appear. After 3–4 months (or two months if the hair grows very quickly) a root retouch relaxer application will be necessary. There will be a clear demarcation line between the previously straightened hair and the new hair growth. It is extremely important to avoid overlapping the relaxer onto the previously straightened hair, as the hair could break. If you should overlap, an orange band may appear on the hair where it has been overprocessed. If you see this, you are too late to prevent damage, so remove the product immediately.

Method for a regrowth application

(1) Prepare the client, scalp, hair and materials. Do not shampoo the hair.
(2) Divide the hair into four equal sections as in Fig. 4.10.
(3) The pattern of application for a regrowth and a virgin application are the same except:

   (a) a tinting brush should be used to apply the product and apply to the demarcation line only, with no overlapping;
   (b) only the area to which the relaxer has been applied should be smoothed.

6.4 Chemical designing

Chemical designing is relaxing hair to create different combinations of straight, wavy and curly hair. It is achieved through a selective and thoughtful chemical application combined with precision cutting and the proper use of conditioners to maintain the hair's body and lustre. Different areas of the head are relaxed more than others to form the intended style. You may use different strengths of relaxer depending on the hair strength and texture. The application will begin at the areas where you want the straightest hair. The relaxer is applied last (or a weaker strength is used) to the areas which require body and movement. An example is shown in Fig. 6.9.

A virgin head of hair is best for chemical designing because previously relaxed hair may have too little support and be too straight for the new hairstyle. It is the degree of relaxation that determines the new hairstyle.

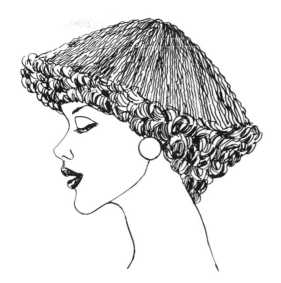

Fig. 6.9 An example of a style created by chemical relaxing (courtesy of TCB).

Relaxing the hair by 50 per cent will reduce the natural curl formation by half. On super-curly hair, this would relax the curl formation into more open curls that could be naturally dried or blow dried straight when desired. A 75 per cent relaxation will leave the hair in a wavy pattern which could be set, blow dried or tonged. A 100 per cent relaxation will completely straighten the hair leaving no visible wave pattern.

An example of chemical designing

Imagine that you want to achieve a look which is smooth on the top with curly support underneath. The relaxer application would begin on the top area where the straightest hair is required (i.e. 85–90 per cent relaxation). The perimeter hair needs relaxing 70–75 per cent so a weaker relaxer would be applied in this area.

After the chemical treatment, the hair is blow dried using more tension on the top hair and less tension on the curly perimeter. Small electric tongs can then be used to curl the ends.

6.5   Home hair-care

Clients seem to learn more about personal hair-care from magazines and television commercials than they do from their hairdressers! They will welcome the expert advice that you are able to offer about looking after their hair between salon visits. Recommend the hair products they need to maintain their style and condition. If possible, display these products in the salon so that your salon increases its turnover rather than giving the profits to the local chemist or supermarket. By following your advice, your clients' hair will look better between salon visits. What could be a better advertisement for your salon than people complimenting your clients about their hair and then asking for the salon's telephone number!

(1) Recommend cleansing, conditioning and styling products and explain what benefits they will have.
(2) Explain how the use of excessive heat and harsh treatment will damage the hair.
(3) Suggest that the hair is covered in excessive sun to protect it from the harmful rays of the sun. Some hair-care products contain built-in sunscreens.
(4) Suggest that clients thoroughly rinse their hair with water after swimming in the sea or in pools treated with chlorine, as both of these make the hair dry.
(5) Explain to the client the necessity to have regular regrowth applications to maintain the style.

6.6   Retail display tips

Do	Don't
Do display all your available stock as a large amount attracts more attention	Don't leave your stock in the stockroom where clients can't see it.
Do make sure that all products are clearly marked with the price.	Don't leave products unpriced because clients may be afraid to ask.
Do make sure that all retail goods are easy to see and accessible.	Don't leave the goods locked up because clients will be reluctant to ask you to take them out.
Do set up your display in busy and waiting areas, e.g. reception.	Don't set up your display where clients cannot see it.
Do make your displays large.	Don't set up too many small ones as they have less impact.
Do use your salon window and entrance area to let passers-by know you sell retail goods.	Don't miss the opportunity to exploit your salon frontage to the full.
Do make your displays attractive and interesting.	Don't use damaged or faded display items.

6.7 Questions

1 What are the two main methods of reducing the amount of curl in hair?
2 Which of these methods is temporary and does not involve the use of chemicals?
3 What form of baldness (alopecia) can occur as a result of using too much tension when pressing hair?
4 What is the name of the bonds which are broken during pressing?
5 Why does sweating of the scalp cause pressed hair to revert back to being curly?
6 What is the difference between a hard and a soft press?
7 Describe how you would carry out a hard press.
8 Why are pressing oils and creams used when carrying out a press?
9 What type of chemical product would you use to relax too much wave in European hair?
10 Describe how you would carry out a relaxing treatment on virgin Afro hair.
11 When relaxing a regrowth, why is it important not to allow the relaxer to come into contact with the previously relaxed hair?
12 Why is it advised to base the scalp before applying a relaxer?
13 What is the name of the amino acid formed, when using a sodium hydroxide type of relaxer, that is not present in virgin hair?
14 Why will you not achieve a good perm result on hair which has been relaxed using a sodium hydroxide type of relaxer?
15 If relaxer is overlapped onto previously relaxed hair when relaxing a regrowth, what could happen?
16 Why should a backwash basin be used for rinsing relaxer out of the hair?
17 If a chemical enters your client's eye what should you do?
18 What advice would you offer your client about home care of relaxed hair?
19 List six important points for the effective display of retail items.

7
Fashion Techniques

Clients are attracted to unusual happenings in the salon, and this attraction can be used to help increase turnover. If your service is unique compared to that offered by your competitors, your clientele will grow. It is like appealing to the person who wants designer clothes rather than those that can be bought from a chain store.

7.1   Introduction

The first part of this chapter will be dealing with the many different ways of winding to achieve interesting results using conventional perming curlers. The second part includes examples of how hair can be permed on other types of 'curlers' or moulds. It is a clear indication that many innovative stylists of today are rejecting perm curlers for more eye-catching methods of winding that can produce sometimes startling results!

In aiming to carry out the perm which will meet the needs of each client, stylists need to select the most appropriate winding technique. For this reason, we have included a range of fashion techniques which show how they are carried out and the type of result they achieve. Fashion winding techniques using conventional perm curlers which are set out in this chapter are:

- *Root perm:* to achieve lift and movement at root area (for short hair only).
- *Texturising (weave perm):* produces variation of curl formation (for short, medium and longer hair).
- *Stack wind:* for curl on perimeter of hair only (for medium to longer hair).
- *Brick wind:* prevents lines in the final perm result (for short, medium and longer hair).
- *Directional wind:* final result falls in direction of the style (for short, medium and longer hair).
- *Twin wind:* produces variation of curl between roots and ends (for medium and longer hair).

Method

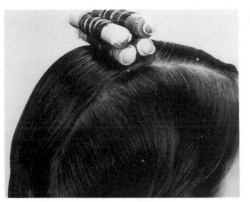

(1) As this winding technique uses twice as many curlers as normal, post-damping is recommended. Winding can therefore begin wherever the stylist chooses. In this case winding begins at the crown. It can clearly be seen how the smaller curler sits on the larger curler which is wound first.

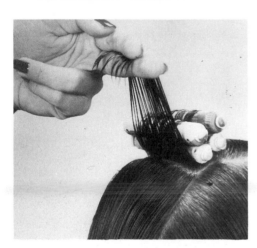

(2) Remember that each mesh should be no longer or wider than the size of the large curler.

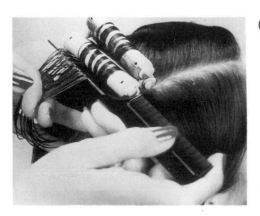

(3) The weaving technique using a pin tail comb. The weaving should be equally spaced. The hair lying over the comb is put out of the way while the strands underneath are wound on the larger curler.

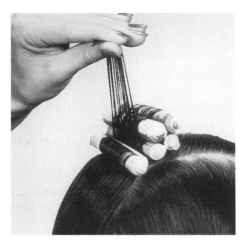

(4) When the larger curler is in position, the remaining strands are then wound on the smaller curler.

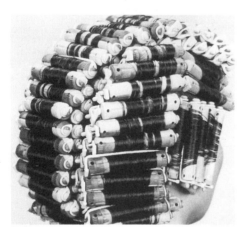

(5) The completed wind ready for damping with the perm lotion.

(Photographs by Wella.)

7.4 Stack wind

A stack wind is the technique used to create a straight effect on top of the head with volume and curl around the perimeter. The curlers are wound to the roots on the underneath hair at the nape and sides to give volume and lift which supports the overlying hair. The placing of the remaining curlers is carefully judged so that each subsequent hair mesh is gradually wound with less hair as you get nearer the crown. Figure 7.2 shows a diagram of a stack wind.

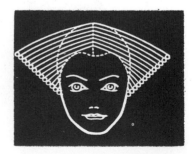

Fig. 7.2 Stack winding.

Winding must begin at the nape so that the overlying hair can be wound and placed in the correct position. In the example that follows, a variation of the stack winding technique is used which gives the hair additional texture because the curlers are wound so that each alternating curler is wound further down the hair than the curlers on either side of it.

Method

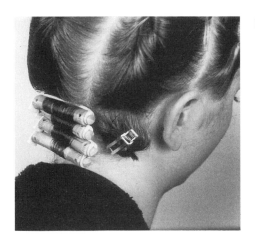

(1) The hair is sectioned into the nine basic sections. It is important to note that winding begins at the *base* of each section, unlike the usual pattern for a basic perm, when winding starts at the top of the section, working downwards.

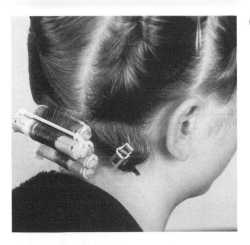

(2) Once you have wound four or five curlers in the normal fashion, right up to the head, it is time to finish your wind a little further away from the roots to achieve less root volume and curl.

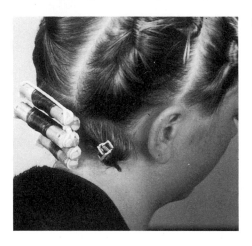

(3) The next curler is wound a little further down to the roots than the last one to achieve a variation in texture.

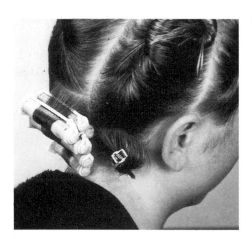

(4) This technique of each alternating curler being wound a little closer to the roots than the preceding one is continuous.

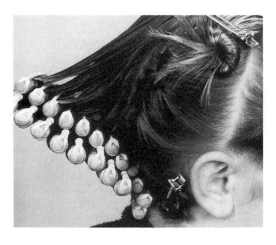

(5) Each curler rests carefully in position on the curler beneath it. Notice how uniformly they are placed and that there is no need for plastic strips slipped through the rubbers to keep them in position.

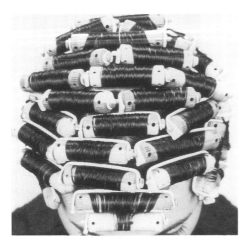

(4) In this example the curlers on the top have been wound forwards and the sides down.

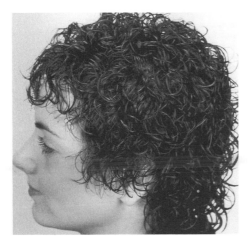

(5) The wet result shows that the hair has no breaks showing any lines caused by placing curlers in straight columns.

(Photographs by Wella.)

7.6 Directional wind

A directional wind is the technique of placing the curlers in the direction of the intended style. This technique helps the hair to maintain its style because it has been permed to lie in a specific direction. The pattern of the wind will depend upon how the hair is to be finally styled. For example, Fig. 7.4 shows the direction of the curlers for a style where the hair is taken over to the side and brought forward onto the face, but a directional wind can be used to encourage

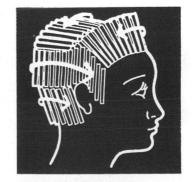

Fig. 7.4 Directional wind.

the hair into whatever direction is required. Normally, directional winds are post-damped, so the winding can begin wherever the stylist chooses.

Method

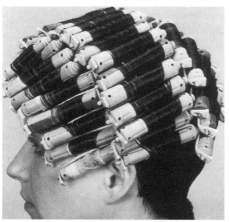

(1)   In this example, winding began at the front hairline directing the curlers to the side from a low parting with the side hair wound downwards.

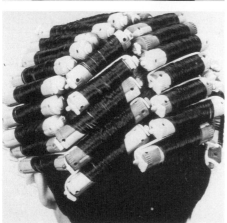

(2)   The back hair has been wound so that it is slightly directed towards the right.

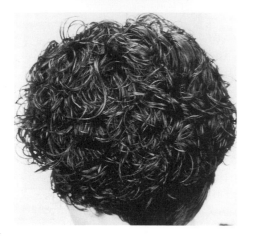

(3)   The wet result shows the natural curl result obtained from using large curlers and carefully planning the pattern that the curlers should be placed in.

(Photographs by Wella.)

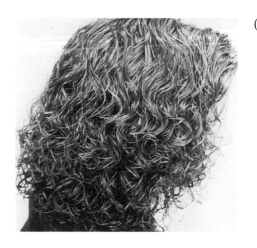

(6) The wet result proves that the twin winding technique creates softer movement on the middle lengths and roots with a stronger curl on the ends.

(Photographs by Wella.)

7.8 Herringbone wind

The herringbone wind is ideal for creating texture in hair without the fear of leaving lines in the final result. The rods are placed so that they resemble the lines of a herringbone instead of in straight lines. This method is suitable for short and medium length hair. In this example, the herringbone winding technique is demonstrated on a male client.

Method

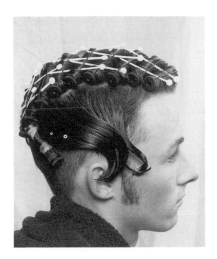

(1) After cleansing with a mild shampoo the hair is towel dried and the client is gowned for a perming service. Winding begins at the front hairline towards the nape and is wound while the hair is damp with water because it will be post-damped. In this case, because the hair is very short around the perimeter (i.e. the nape and sides), the winding finishes in the occipital region. End papers are used to prevent buckled ends; notice how smoothly the hair is wrapped around each rod.

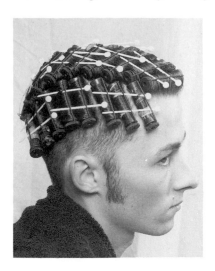

(2) Plastic setting pins or 'picks' have been used to take the stress off the hair where the elastic fasteners rest on the hair. Even if the elastic fasteners are round in shape and not too tight, stress marks can appear on the hair. Do not use metal pins to do this as they can react with the perm lotion.

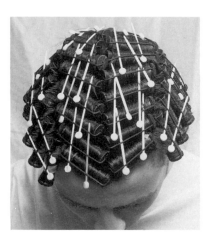

(3) Here you can clearly see the top view of the wind showing how the placing of the rods resembles herringbone lines. This picture also shows how the plastic pins relieve any stress which might have otherwise been put on the hair by the elastic fasteners of the rods. Now that winding is complete, the stylist would now place a cotton wool strip around the outside of the wound rods to protect the client's skin during the application of the perm lotion. After the perm lotion is applied, the perm is developed according to the manufacturer's instructions. When the hair is sufficiently processed, the hair is then neutralised following the manufacturer's instructions.

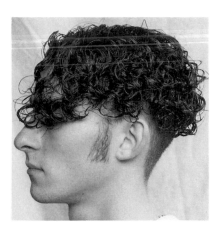

(4) This shows the final wet result which can be left to dry naturally or gently scrunch-dried with a hair drier for a fuller effect. Notice how natural the curl formation is and how there are no marks or separation lines where the rods were placed.

(Photographs by Zotos (UK) Ltd.)

7.9 Spiral wind

The spiral wind is used on long hair to ensure that the curl formation is equal along the hair shaft from roots to points. If the rods were placed horizontally on such long hair, the curl result would be weaker at the roots because each time the mesh of hair is wrapped around the rod, the circumference of the rod is gradually increasing because the hair is wrapped so many times over itself. This increase in the circumference of the rod does not happen during spiral winding.

Method

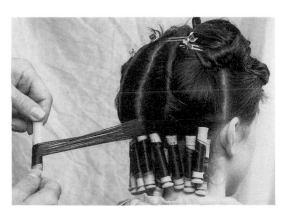

(1) After cleansing with a mild shampoo, the hair is towel dried and sectioned into four main divisions by making partings from the forehead to nape and across the top of the head from ear to ear. If there is to be a side parting, adjust the parting at the centre of the top of the head to its correct position. The hair will be post-damped so is wound while the hair is damp with water. As the picture shows, winding starts at the nape and works upwards. Sections which are approximately one centimetre

square are used starting at the centre of the head and winding the hair in an outward direction towards the face. Notice that the hair is positioned onto the rod at the lower end so the hair is only overlapped onto itself by 50 per cent.

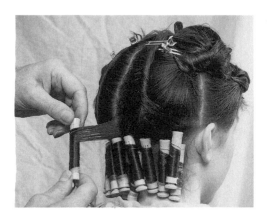

(2) It is very important to limit this overlap to 50 per cent otherwise the curl formation will be weaker where the overlap exceeds this. The picture shows that it is necessary to use the entire length of the rod when winding in this way.

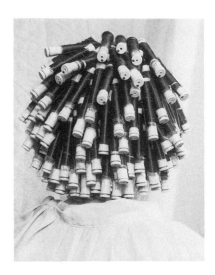

(3) The wind continues using one centimetre square sections up towards the crown. This shows the view of the completed wind at the back of the head.

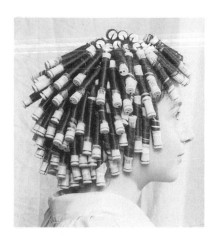

(4) The sides are wound in the same way by staring at the bottom of the front sections and working upwards towards the middle or side parting. In this example the client wears a side parting and the hair has been wound to take this into account.

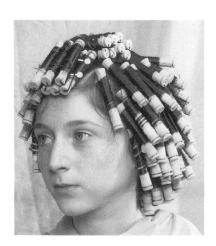

(5) This shows the other side of the head and the side parting is clearly visible. To create maximum lift and texture at the front, the hair is wound away from the side parting using the double wrap winding technique. Plastic pins have been used on the rods at the front to avoid any pressure marks being caused by the elastic fasteners. The hair is now ready to have the perm lotion applied and be developed according to the manufacturer's instructions. After the recommended development time, a curl test is taken to monitor the degree of curl which has been formed and to check if the hair is ready for neutralising.

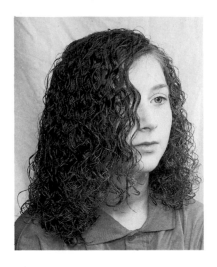

(6)   The picture shows the hair after neutralising and the wet result which has been achieved. You can see how even the curl formation is along the hair length and the added lift to the roots of the hair at the side parting where the hair was wound using the double wrap technique. The hair could now be left to dry naturally or gently scrunch-dried with a hair drier to achieve a more voluminous effect.

(Photographs by Zotos (UK) Ltd.)

ALTERNATIVE WINDING TECHNIQUES

7.10   Tissue perming

Tissue perming is a winding technique which uses tissues instead of perm curlers as a mould. It can be used on short or long hair and is ideal for fragile hair, when a lot of movement is required as there is no undue strain on the hair from the rubbers or pins. It is best to use a box of multicoloured tissues because they will be an eye-catcher in the salon. Do be careful, however, of using green tissues on blonde hair as the colour may bleed and stain the hair!

To prepare the tissues, fold them in half diagonally to make a triangle. Begin rolling up the tissue starting at the point to form a narrow 'sausage'. Now twist the tissue to make it rigid.

How is a tissue perm carried out?

(1)   Shampoo and towel dry the hair. Apply a pre-perm treatment if the hair is porous.

(2)   Section the hair in triangles; for a loose movement use large sections, for a tighter movement use small sections. Dampen each section of hair thoroughly as you wind. Use an end paper to keep the points of the hair in place and wind the hair the same way as you would if using conventional curlers. To secure the tissue in place, tie the ends together in a knot. For a spiral curl result, hold the tissue vertically and spiral wind the hair around it.

(3)   Do not use a plastic cap to cover the tissues during processing. When processing is complete, *do not rinse the hair* or the tissues will disintegrate!

(4) Use two to three times more neutraliser than normal and carefully saturate each tissue. Continue neutralising as normal, and remove the tissues, which will now be breaking up, after about five minutes. Rinse and condition the hair.

(5) Proceed with styling as usual.

7.11 *Molton Brown perm*

Molton Brown permers (also called Molton permers) can be used to carry out a basic wind instead of using conventional perm curlers. There is no tight band on the bendy permer to keep it in position; instead, the ends of the permer are bent back just beside the edges of the wound hair which hold it comfortably in place. These permers are very much lighter than the heavier conventional perm curlers because they are made of foam and are often preferred by clients because they are more comfortable.

Method

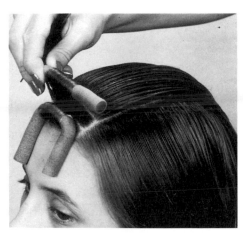

(1) As this technique can be post-damped, winding can begin wherever the stylist chooses. In this example, the stylist has chosen to begin at the front hairline. Meshes are taken the same width as the diameter of the permer being used. When the permer is wound down to the root the ends are bent back to keep it in place.

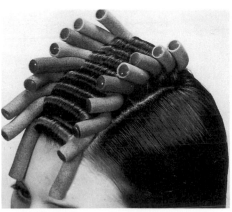

(2) In this example the basic wind pattern is followed, winding the hair straight back from the front hairline.

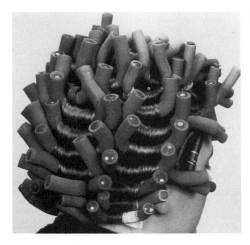

(3) The permers follow the same pattern as a basic wind except at the sides where the hair is wound forward towards the face. All the permers rest firmly in position while being very comfortable for the client.

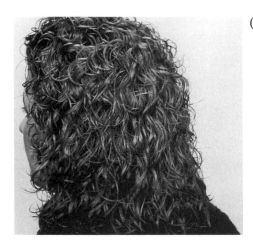

(4) The wet result. There is a soft curl movement without a bandmark in sight!

(Photographs by Wella.)

7.12   Spiral wind using Molton permers

The ideal technique for creating a spiral curl result is using Molton permers with a spiral wind. The meshes of hair are held vertically and are wound and twisted around the permer. These permers come in two lengths and three widths. This means that long hair can be spirally wound because you can choose the permer size that will allow the hair to be wound up evenly all the way up to the roots.

Method

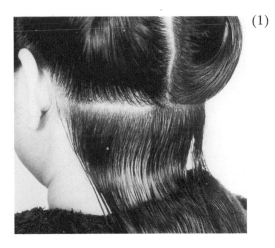

(1) Winding should begin at the nape so that the unwound hair can be neatly kept out of the way. The best method for sectioning is to divide the hair into two at the back and clip it out of the way, leaving a section of hair approximately 4 cms (1½ inches) deep, as shown.

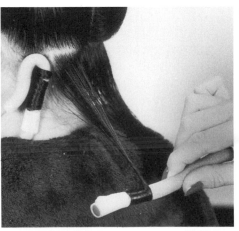

(2) Begin winding by taking a section about 2 cms wide (almost an inch). Wrap the hair around the permer (using a perm paper) with the points positioned slightly to one end of the permer to make maximum use of its length. This can be seen in the picture. At this stage the permer is held horizontally.

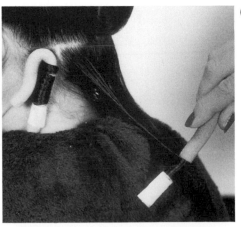

(3) As the hair is wound the hands turn the permer through 360° to create a twist in the hair. The twisting is done several times as the hair is wound up to the root. Notice that the permer is now held vertically.

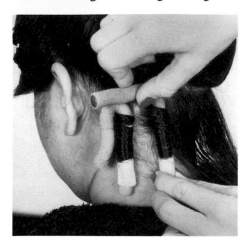

(4) Once the permer is wound down to the roots, the end is bent downwards to hold it in position.

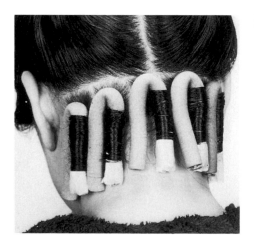

(5) The completed first section. To continue winding, another section about 4 cms wide is parted off across the back of the head and the permers are wound in the same fashion. Winding continues in the same manner over the whole head, but remember to begin the winding on the underneath hair at the sides, the same as the back.

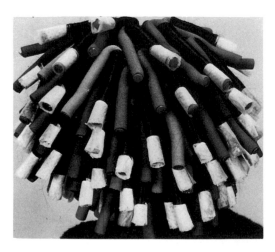

(6) The completed wind. No pins or clips are needed to keep the permers in place.

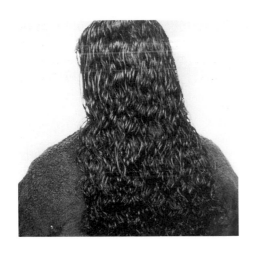

(7) The wet result. The movement goes right to the root, and the curl is open and falls spirally.

(Photographs by Wella.)

7.13 Mad Mats

At the Mad Hackers Hair Asylum salon in London, Maureen and Kevin Bura have revolutionised perming by designing a new hairdressing tool which they call Mad Mats. The product looks like a J-Cloth and has fine wires running through foam and material. Mad Mats are reusable and come in three widths and lengths. They are available to other hairdressers from Mad Hackers.

- Size 1 – pink (the largest)
- Size 2 – yellow
- Size 3 – blue

Mad Mats can be used for setting or perming, and successful techniques used by Mad Hackers include root perming, spiral perming, zig-zag and straightening. The hair can be curled, twisted, and even corrugated because Mad Mats can be easily manipulated into any shape. No end papers or pins are needed and they are particularly good for perming woven cut hair (which is difficult to perm on curlers because of the varying lengths) as they give the stylist complete control of the hair meshes. Because they are light, clients find this technique more comfortable than perms done with conventional curlers.

How are Mad Mats used?

A mesh of hair is placed on the Mat which is then folded over to hold the hair in place. Once the Mat is in place, manipulate it into the shape that will give you the result you want to achieve. If you want a crimped look, corrugate the Mat; if you want a soft, spiral curl, twist the hair round the full length of the Mat. Choose whatever perm lotion and neutraliser suits the hair texture and process as usual. Mad Hackers suggest that if the hair is short, apply the perm lotion as you wind, but if it is long, apply the lotion after winding is complete. Care should be taken to ensure that the hair is completely saturated.

Step-by-step to achieving the zig-zag effect

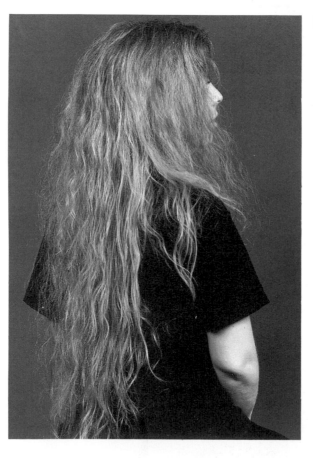

(1) Long, naturally wavy hair is shampooed and excess moisture is removed to leave the hair damp.

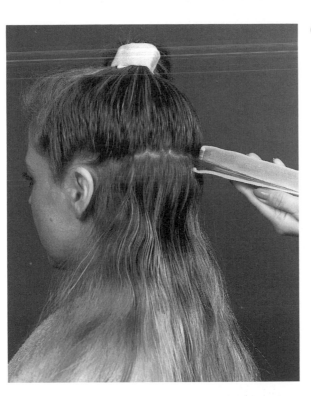

(2) The hair is divided so that the back, underneath hair is wound first. A mesh of hair is taken and the Mat is folded in half lengthways, over the hair.

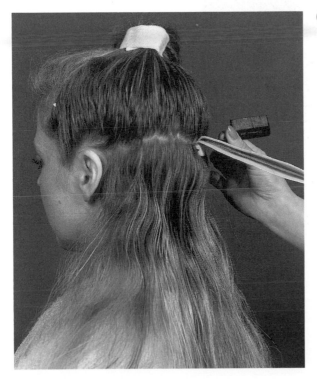

(3) The end of the tail comb is used to make a crease at the root which will hold the Mat securely in place.

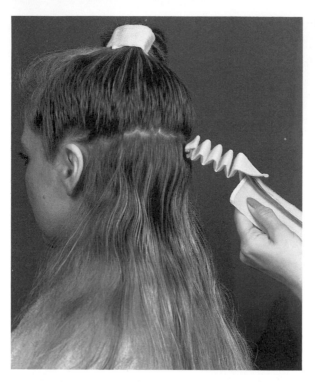

(4)   The Mat is bent into a zig-zag using the end of the tail comb. As this hair is very long, a second Mat is joined to the first so that all the hair can be wound.

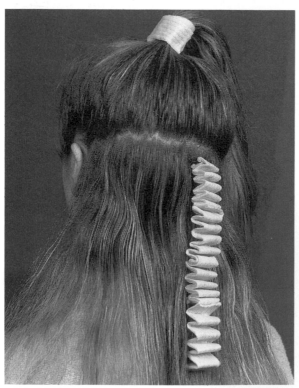

(5)   Use as many Mats as are needed to wind the length of the mesh, ensuring that the zig-zag is equally proportional. Continue winding the rest of the hair in this way.

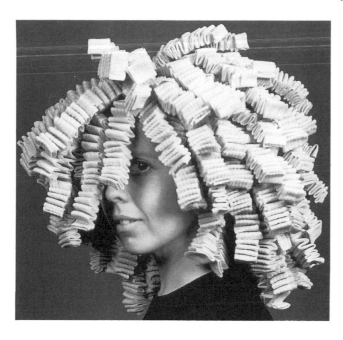

(6) The completed wind showing just what an eye-catcher this would be in the salon!

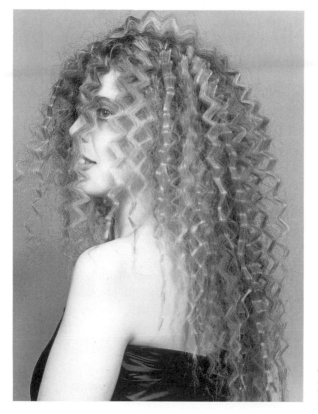

(7) The finished result shows the zig-zag form that has been created in the hair.

(Photographs courtesy of Mad Hackers Hair Asylum.)

Note: Similar effects can be produced using aluminium foil instead of Mad Mats.

7.14   Tint tube perm

This perming technique achieves an angular wave in the hair using flat, rectangular-shaped flexible 'curlers'. To make one of these curlers, take an empty tint tube and cut off both ends. Flatten the tube, clean it and cover it with foil (no chemical reaction will occur with the chemicals in perming systems). The curler is secured by bending the ends inwards, so no pins are necessary. Different rod widths are achieved by cutting the tint tube lengthways.

How is a tint perm carried out?

(1)   Shampoo and towel dry the hair. Apply a pre-perm treatment if the hair is porous.
(2)   Wind in the direction of the finished style, choosing the width of curler that will achieve the desired degree of movement. The narrower curlers will produce a tighter movement. Make your meshes slightly narrower than the length of the curler as the ends will be folded inwards to secure it in place. Use end papers to keep the ends of the hair together and in place.
(3)   Hair can be wound with or without lotion. When winding is completed, saturate each curler with lotion and leave to process. Process and neutralise as directed by the manufacturers of the product you are using.
(4)   To finish, ruffle the hair with the fingers and allow it to dry naturally. Do not comb the hair or you will destroy the angular shape. Advise the client that they should only comb their hair before shampooing.

7.15   Rik-Rak winding

Rik-Raks are flexible plastic curlers which are V-shaped. They come in different lengths and achieve the same deep zig-zag wave created by plaiting wet hair, and then releasing it when it is dry. Meshes of hair are woven through the two arms of the curler in a figure of eight. The hair should not be twisted during winding and the tension should be kept even. Rik-Raks can be used for setting or perming hair.

How is a Rik-Rak wind carried out?

(1)   Shampoo and towel dry the hair. Apply a pre-perm treatment if the hair is porous.

(2) Begin winding at the nape taking square sections no larger than 3 cms (just over 1 inch).

(3) Use an end paper on the points of the hair and wind for 2–3 turns on a small diameter perm curler.

(4) Place the hair between the two arms of the Rik-Rak and weave a figure of eight, as in Fig. 7.6.

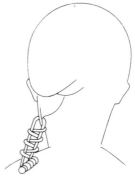

Fig. 7.6

(5) Continue working towards the crown. Try to work in a brick formation so that the curlers rest between one another. This will help to balance the curls evenly and prevent breaks in the final dressing. The curler does not have to be placed right at the root. For a smooth crown area leave the roots free as in Fig. 7.7. Wind the sides in the same way.

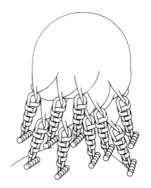

Fig. 7.7

(6) When the winding is complete, saturate each curler with the perm lotion. Process the hair without a plastic cap. To check development of the perm, gently unravel a little of the hair to judge the depth of wave.

(7) Rinse and neutralise in the usual way. (You can, however, leave the curlers in place after the final rinse for drying provided that you have allowed the full neutraliser development time.)

(8) After final rinsing and conditioning, continue with styling. If you decide to leave the curlers in place for drying, gently brush the hair to create body and volume.

7.16 Pincurl perm

Using pincurls for perming can create directional movement in the hair with or without lift at the root. Using pincurls at the sides and nape areas is the ideal method for achieving soft directional movement when no root lift is required. Pincurls can easily be incorporated into many style winds when the rest of the hair is wound on curlers.

It is very important that the pincurls are perfect as any incorrect movement will, of course, be permanent! Use plastic clips to prevent any reaction between the perm lotion and metal clips. Cotton wool can be used to pad the pincurls to prevent them from collapsing. Any type of pincurl can be used depending on the result you want to achieve. Here are some guidelines to the types of pincurls you could use and their effects:

Figure 7.8. Open pincurl. An open pincurl will give you a soft movement.

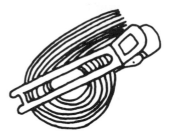

Fig. 7.8

Figure 7.9. Closed pincurl. A closed pincurl will give you a stronger curl movement which will be tighter at the points than an open pincurl.

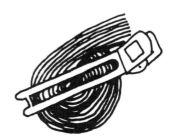

Fig. 7.9

Figure 7.10. Stand-up pincurl. A stand-up pincurl will give you root lift. This type of pincurl will require padding to prevent it from collapsing during the perming process.

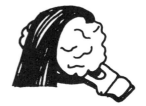

Fig. 7.10

How is a pincurl perm carried out?

(1) Shampoo and towel dry the hair. Apply a pre-perm treatment if the hair is porous. Pincurl perms can be wound with the lotion or post-damped.
(2) As the pincurls will probably be wound in the direction of the client's natural hair growth pattern, begin making your pincurls wherever you find it easiest (most stylists begin at the front hairline). Make your pincurls on even sections about 2 cms (just less than an inch) square.

The larger the square base is for your pincurl, the larger the curl movement will be at the root. Remember to pad any pincurls that might collapse with cotton wool or crêpe hair. If you have difficulty with the points of the hair, try using a small piece of an end paper or crêpe hair to help hold them together and in place.

(3)   When you have completed your wind, apply the perm lotion if you have wound without lotion, or re-damp the pincurls with lotion if you have pre-damped.

(4)   Allow the perm to process according to the manufacturer's instructions and the type of hair you are working with. If possible, avoid the use of a plastic cap as it could disturb your pincurls.

(5)   After processing, gently place a fine setting net over the client's head to minimise disturbance to the pincurls. Use the water on a low pressure and take extra care while neutralising in the usual way.

(6)   After neutralising, apply a conditioner. The hair is now ready for further styling.

7.17   The chopstick perm

Perming the hair using chopsticks was pioneered by a Chinese hairdresser, Alan Soh, in London. He perfected the skill of winding hair around chopsticks to produce uniform and resilient ringlets, and has held many seminars to teach other hairdressers this skill.

Using chopsticks has four main features:

- Very long hair can be permed because the length of a chopstick allows the mesh to be wrapped evenly. Using conventional perm curlers on long hair usually results in the hair falling off the end, creating an uneven result.
- Because the hair is wound around the chopstick spirally (i.e. from root to points) with no overlap, the resultant curl is completely uniform in formation throughout its entire length. When using ordinary perm curlers, the hair is wound over itself many times on long hair which makes the curl looser near the roots.
- There are no rubber bands to damage the hair because the chopstick is secured with a pin at the roots and a pipe cleaner is used to hold the points in position.
- It is a real eye-catcher in the salon and helps to promote perming.

Method

(1)   Shampoo and towel dry the hair.
(2)   Divide the hair from forehead to nape down the centre.

(3) A section of hair is divided off at the nape which is approximately 6 cms (2½ inches) deep. The remaining hair should be clipped neatly out of the way.

(4) This section is then divided so that meshes of hair approximately 4 cms (1½ inches) wide are wound on the chopsticks (see Fig. 7.11).

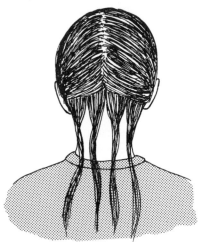

Fig. 7.11 Chopstick winding begins at the nape, using sections that are approximately 6 cms × 4 cms.

(5) Each mesh is dampened with the perm lotion before it is wound. The chopstick is held in the right hand and the left hand winds the mesh securely around it. This is shown in Fig. 7.12. A pipe cleaner (cut into 5 cm lengths) is used to hold the points securely in place on the chopstick. To secure the chopstick at the roots, the chopstick is turned a full 360 degrees a couple of times to ensure the roots will also have movement in the final result. An ordinary setting pin is then pushed through the twisted roots and this will hold the chopstick firmly in position.

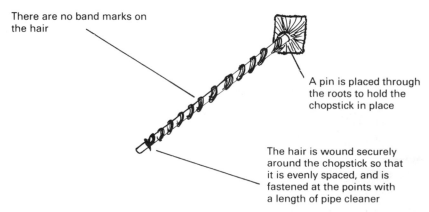

There are no band marks on the hair

A pin is placed through the roots to hold the chopstick in place

The hair is wound securely around the chopstick so that it is evenly spaced, and is fastened at the points with a length of pipe cleaner

Fig. 7.12 A wound mesh is secured onto the chopstick.

(6)   Once all the meshes have been wound in this section, another section is taken and the winding continues. When the top of the head is reached, it is recommended that triangular sections be taken instead of straight ones to prevent straight lines appearing in the finished look.

(7)   When all the hair is wound it must be covered with a plastic cap. As an ordinary perm cap will be too small to fit over the chopsticks, a clean plastic refuse bag is used. It can be split down one side and held in position with clips.

(8)   The hair should be processed and neutralised in the usual manner. The chopsticks can be easily removed and more neutraliser should then be applied.

(9)   The new perm should not be combed or brushed as this will disturb the perfectly uniform ringlets that you have created. Leave the hair to dry naturally under infra-red heaters (Climazon, octopus lamps).

(10)   If you so desire, gently loosen the curl by 'combing' through gently with two chopsticks; this creates a softer look. Using chopsticks works equally well for the setting of hair. You could promote this as a special look for brides with long hair.

7.18   Sellotape perm

A sellotape perm is used to create maximum lift at the roots and straight unpermed middle lengths and ends. A sellotape perm is best used in conjunction with other winding techniques for a multi-textured look, although it can be used by itself for specific designs.

To increase the amount of overall root lift which can be achieved by the root perming method, the sellotape technique can be used in the areas where increased lift is required, by alternating between a perm curler and sellotape.

Method

(1)   Wind the hair using the root perm technique according to the intended style but leave out a mesh of hair between two curlers in the places or areas where you want to achieve the increased root volume. Once the winding is complete you will be left with meshes of hair left unwound between some (or all) of the curlers.

(2)   Divide each of these meshes into two equal parts. Twist one of the strands in a clockwise direction until it is tightly coiled. Twist the other strand in the opposite direction (i.e. anticlockwise). Without letting go of the twisted strands, wrap the middle lengths and ends with the sellotape so that they are covered with a plastic 'film'.

(3) Process and neutralise the perm as usual. You will find the sellotape easy to remove because it softens once it is rinsed with the warm water during the neutralising procedure.

(4) The meshes which are permed using the sellotape technique will stand out from the head. Because the middle lengths were protected by the sellotape, these parts will remain unprocessed and thus create more texture throughout the finished look.

> Remember, it is *only* your skill and imagination that restricts how you choose to perm hair. Hairdressers have been known to perm hair using coat hangers, pipe cleaners and even match boxes! Plastic hair-dividing clips have been used to hold scrunched hair in position for perming. Experiment and enjoy your work – perming can be fun!

7.19   Questions

1   What is a root perm?
2   Why are two different sizes of curler used in texturising?
3   When would you use a stack wind?
4   What type of hair would you use a brick wind on?
5   What is the advantage of this type of wind?
6   What is a directional wind?
7   For what type of result would you use twin winding?
8   What is a tissue perm?
9   Why should green tissues be avoided on blonde hair?
10   When would you use a herringbone wind?
11   What is the advantage of using Molton Browners?
12   How would you wind a spiral perm?
13   Describe Mad Mats and what you might use them for.
14   How would you prepare tint tubes for a tint tube perm?
15   How would you secure the tint tubes in place?
16   What are Rik-Raks?
17   When would you use pincurls for a perm?
18   Describe how you would section the hair for a chopstick perm.
19   How is the hair secured on the chopstick?
20   Can you think of at least one new winding technique?

8
History

8.1 Perming

The permanent curling of straight hair is by no means a new idea. It goes back as far as the early Egyptians who wound their hair on sticks, coated it with mud, and then baked it in the sun.

About four hundred years ago, European wigmakers produced permanent curl in the hair they used to make wigs and hairpieces. They wound the hair on sticks and boiled it in water for at least thirty minutes. This technique is still used today, and is called *frizzure forcée* by wigmakers. Obviously, this method could not be used on live people who had to make do with pin sets and hot irons to produce the curls and waves that they desired.

It was not until the beginning of the twentieth century that a method of perming was introduced that could be safely used on people. This method involved the use of heat and was therefore known as 'heat perming'. Heat perming was used widely in many different forms until the end of the Second World War, some systems still being used in salons as late as the 1950s.

Heat perming systems were time-consuming and complex operations. This also made them expensive and restricted their use to the rich. First, the hair was divided into small square sections over the entire head. Using a special hook, the hair in each section was twisted and pulled through a rubber square (with a hole in it) which was pushed down close to the scalp. This rubber provided a protective layer between the scalp and the heat on every square section. The section of hair (which was at this stage protruding through the rubber protector) was then wound from root to point and secured with string. Then either a borax paste was applied to the hair, or a special sachet (consisting of tissue paper and an absorbent pad

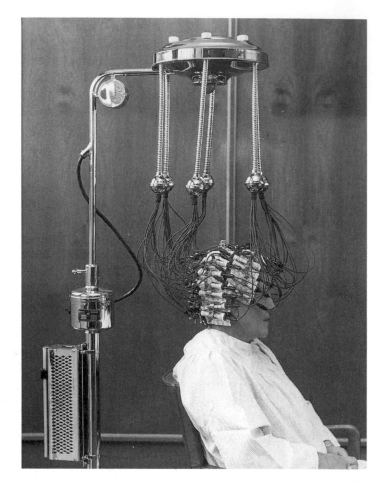

Fig. 8.1   Wella-Rapid Hot Permanent Waving Machine (reproduced courtesy of Wella).

dipped into an ammonia solution) was wrapped around the wound hair. Muslin, flannel, paper or gauze would then be used to cover and protect the hair. Some perm systems had special metal clips used to fasten the wound curler at the roots to prevent steam escaping and burning the scalp. Heat would then be applied using special heaters. An example of such a machine is shown in Fig. 8.1. (This is a later, more sophisticated model.) Each wound curler was inserted into a heater for processing. These heaters were heavy and cumbersome, and many clients found the experience of being wired up to a machine worrying. In the event of an air-raid occurring halfway through the process, the client was often left alone in the salon, still attached to the machine! After processing for between one and fifteen minutes, the hair was allowed to cool before removing the curlers. The hair could then be gently shampooed and set.

The early type of heat perming machines caused discomfort to the client because they produced mild electric shocks and scalp burns. The excessive heat which was used also caused very dry hair. Because the curlers used at this time were narrow, the perms were always tight and lasted a long time. Clients would have probably had only two perms a year, allowing the previous one to be completely removed by cutting before the next perm.

This type of perming system is usually credited to a German hairdresser, Karl Nessler. In Fig. 8.2, Nessler (centre) is seen demonstrating his ideas to the two Ströher brothers, the founders of Wella. It is thought that about 1910, Nessler, E. Frederics and Eugene Suter, all working independently of each other, discovered that the addition of borax to hot water gave a curl that lasted several washings. About 1924, ammonium hydroxide was used in conjunction with borax to give a more lasting curl.

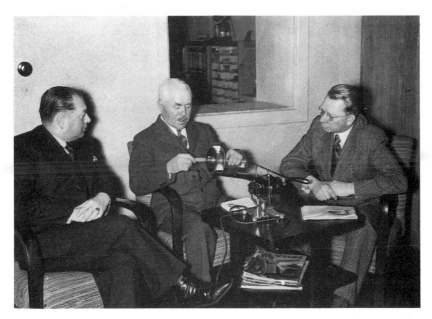

Fig. 8.2 Nessler (the father of permanent waving) is seated centre, demonstrating his latest inventions to the Ströher brothers in 1937 (reproduced courtesy of Wella).

The Wella-Rapid hot perming machine was introduced about 1932; an advertisement from the trade magazine *Hairdresser's Weekly Journal* is shown in Fig. 8.3 featuring the machine. Notice that it boasts a time of 65 minutes! Also, you can see that a low voltage was used to lessen the risks of electric shock! This type of machine used lower temperatures and milder reagents. The actual curler contained an element which was connected to the curler contacts on the machine to provide the heat. The hair was then

WELLA-RAPID
The Permanent Waving Machine which brings Prosperity to your Business

LOW VOLTAGE:
Steaming on 24 volts.

FALLING HEAT:
Simmering on 16 volts.

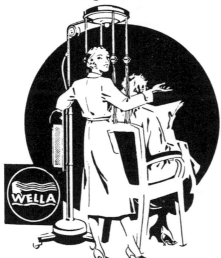

ABSOLUTE SAFETY. NO RISK OF BURNING OR SCALDING.

SIMPLICITY ITSELF.

Ideal for those about to commence Permanent Waving.

The most Rapid System in existence. A beautiful Permanent Wave with tight clinging curls in approx. **65** minutes.

TIME SAVING AND MONEY MAKING

Special Trade Demonstrations
arranged in

GLASGOW GRAND HOTEL, CHARING CROSS

Tuesday, May 16th, Wednesday, May 17th, and Thursday, May 18th, at 11 a.m., 3 p.m., 5 p.m. and 7 p.m. on each day.

To be held under the auspices of our Scottish Agent, MR. E. GODFREY.

MODELS FROM 31 GNS. TO £77

BE SURE OF SUCCESS AND INSTAL THE MODERN SYSTEM

Fig. 8.3   An advertisement for the Wella-Rapid machine in a 1933 edition of *Hairdresser's Weekly Journal* (reproduced courtesy of Wella).

wound from points to roots (called the *croquignole* winding method) as opposed to the spiral winding technique which involved winding from roots to points. The croquignole winding technique was quicker to do and the curler contacts connected to the element in the curler at each end were not as heavy. Figure 8.1 actually shows a client attached to a Wella-Rapid machine.

The next breakthrough was the introduction of wireless, machineless

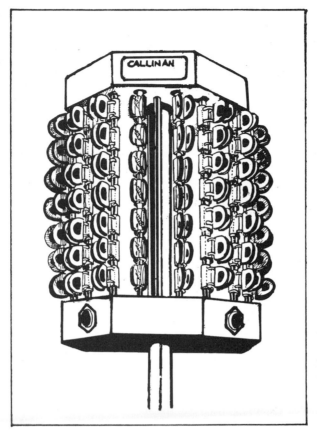

Fig. 8.4 The Callinan Machine.

perming systems. They were at their height in the 1940s, and had the advantage that there was no risk of electric shock and the client had freedom of head movement.

The Callinan perming system used metal clamps, which were heated on the bars of an electric unit like the one shown in Fig. 8.4. The hair was first divided into small squares over the entire head and each mesh was slipped through a rubber scalp protector using a hook. The hair was then saturated with a sulphur-based solution before being wound in croquignole fashion on a special metal curler. As end papers had not yet been introduced, crêpe hair was used to prevent buckled ends. (Crêpe hair is made from hair which has been permanently curled by boiling and baking, and thus has a wiry texture.) The metal curler was wound with the help of a special handle which was inserted into one end of the curler. Several sizes of curler were available which could all be fitted into the Callinan handle, making the wind easier and faster. A Callinan curler in its handle is shown in Fig. 8.5. Once each individual curler was wound, the heated clamp was placed over the curler and the handle was removed, leaving the wound

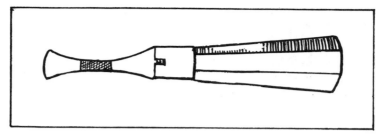

Fig. 8.5 A Callinan curler in handle.

curler in position. There were two sizes of heated clamps available to suit the size of the curlers used. After sufficient processing, the clamps were removed and the hair was allowed to cool before shampooing and setting the hair.

Also in the 1940s, a tepid perming system was introduced that did not require the use of a machine. An example of this type of perm is the Jamal system. The hair was sectioned into the same nine sections that are used today for basic winds. There was no specific order of winding because the hair would not process until the special exothermic sachet was applied. For this reason, most hairdressers began winding at the front as it was easier. A narrow mesh of hair was taken and slipped through a rubber scalp protector. A special metal clamp was then placed at the root, close to the rubber protector, and the hair was evenly spread along the opening, as shown in Fig. 8.6. The clamp was then fastened and the correct strength lotion applied. The Jamal lotions were available in three strengths:

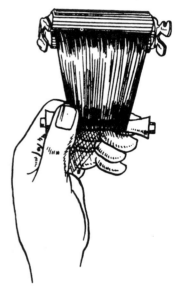

Fig. 8.6 Hair being wound down onto a clamp. The grip is altered as the winding proceeds.

Lotion 1 – fine hair
Lotion 2 – coarse hair
Lotion 3 – tinted hair

To prevent buckled ends, crêpe hair was used on the points of the hair, because the croquignole winding technique was used. Careful positioning of the hands was very important during winding to ensure that the correct angle was achieved for an even and smooth wind. After all the hair was wound, the exothermic sachets were dipped into water and then squeezed out before being applied to the individual curlers. These sachets, first used in England in 1923, contained calcium oxide (quicklime). Once wet, this turned into calcium hydroxide (slaked lime) with the evolution of a great deal of heat, activating the lotion on the hair. An exothermic chemical reaction is one which gives off heat. The sachets expanded during the reaction and had to be held in place with special clips. Once the sachet had cooled, the curlers were removed and the hair was shampooed and set. At this point, it would be appropriate to consider the chemistry of heat perming.

Chemistry of heat perming

Figure 8.7 shows the hair in its natural straight state, containing disulphide bonds.

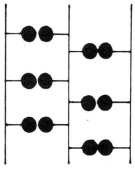

Fig. 8.7

Key to Figs 8.7–8.10

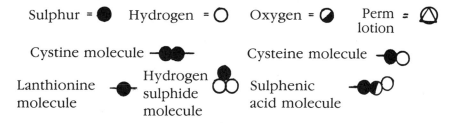

In Fig. 8.8 the hair is saturated with lotion (containing ammonium hydroxide, borax and sodium sulphite) and is then wound onto curlers. No reaction occurs until heat is applied to the curlers.

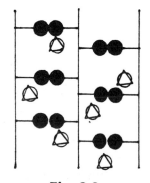

Fig. 8.8

In Fig. 8.9 heat has been applied to the curler and two types of chemical reaction occur. Some disulphide bonds are broken by *reduction* as in cold waving (the sulphite works at temperatures above 60°C). Most of the bonds are broken by *hydrolysis* (the chemical addition of water). Cystine is broken down to *sulphenic acid* and *cysteine*.

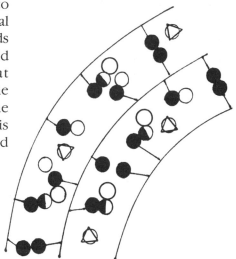

Fig. 8.9

In Fig. 8.10 the sulphenic acid and cysteine molecules have joined to form the amino acid *lanthionine*, which has only one sulphur. Water and hydrogen sulphide gas (rotten eggs smell) are given off as this happens. The hair is then rinsed and set.

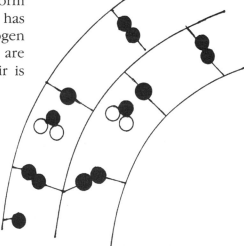

Fig. 8.10

Towards the end of the 1930s the first cold permanent waving systems were being produced, based on thioglycollic acid. Because of the Second World War their development was slowed up. Chemists and chemicals were being used for other purposes!

In the 1940s and 1950s the cold wave was improved. The product used after the War was harsh compared to that of today, but was available in different strengths for different hair types. The hair was wound in the basic nine sections using curlers which would be classified as small by today's standards. The results were tight and lasting, but there was often an unpleasant smell of ammonia in the hair for a while afterwards.

Each change in fashion influences the way that hair is styled. While perming hair might be the vogue one season, colour may become all-important the next season. Perming systems are now available for almost all hair types and the techniques developed allow the texture of hair to be changed into a variety of curls, waves, spirals and even zig-zags. But we are still winding the hair onto a curler or mould, in much the same way as the ancient Egyptians.

Today's trend is towards less alkaline perm lotions. In future editions of this book we might well have to talk about cold waves as a thing of the past. A few years ago, the idea of an acid perm would have been regarded as impossible because it was assumed that alkalinity was necessary to allow penetration through the cuticle into the cortex. Perhaps some revolutionary products are being developed at this very moment. The day may come when you can take a pill to alter your natural hair growth so it changes from straight to curly. Who knows?

8.2   *Straightening and relaxing*

The slaves from Africa who began to arrive in Europe and the Americas from the mid-seventeenth century onwards had no use for the typical comb used by white people. It was impossible to draw the comb through their tight, curly hair, because the teeth of the comb were too closely set together. They made their own crude combs from farm implements which had long teeth, widely spaced apart – the forerunner to the Afro comb of today.

The effect of existing in a totally different environment, where their rich masters had straight hair, influenced the way that they wore their hair. Instead of wearing it naturally curly, or plaiting and braiding it into exotic styles, the hair was worn straight. They would pack axle grease into their hair and then brush it until it was straight. Soap was used to remove the axle grease from the hair. Eventually, the build-up of such heavy grease made the scalp feel very sore. When the scalp became too painful to endure, the hair would be cut off and once the scalp was healthy again, the process would begin again.

In the last century, temporary straightening of the hair was achieved by a heated metal tool or rod being stroked over the hair. The hair was also wrapped in pieces of cloth and pressed using a flattened, heated can. Temporary waves were obtained by wrapping wet hair in rags tied with string. They would sleep with the rags in their hair and the following day would have waves. Hot irons were also used to press the hair and to create straight line crimps. It was not until 1872 that a French hairdresser named Marcel Grateau revolutionised the use of hot irons by developing a series of movements which created waves. Up until that time, the irons were used in a way that could only produce straight line crimps. Hence such irons are often referred to as Marcel irons (Fig. 8.11).

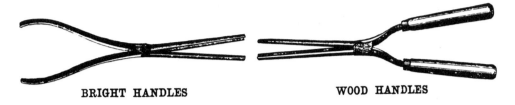

BRIGHT HANDLES   WOOD HANDLES

Fig. 8.11 Marcel waving irons.

Around 1900, pressing combs, such as the one shown in Fig. 8.12 became popular. These were heated over a flame and then drawn through the hair repeatedly until it was straight. Scalp burns were a frequent occurrence, and the hair became dry from the excessive use of heat. To improve the hair's condition a number of remedies were used, including castor oil, eggs and rainwater.

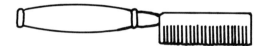

Fig. 8.12 Pressing comb.

During the 1920s the 'flapper' girl emerged with shorter skirts, belted hips, and a hairstyle called 'the bob'. The original bobs were flat, short and had fringes. This was a difficult style to maintain using the temporary straightening methods. It was around this time that the first recipes for permanent hair relaxers were introduced which were a mixture of lye, lard and petroleum jelly. Serious scalp burns and hair loss were common because the mixture was strong and an application technique had not yet been perfected.

Gradually, over the years, lye-based relaxing creams were developed, incorporating improved conditioning agents. Acid rinses also helped to reduce damage. The advent of the thioglycollic acids for cold perms soon resulted in the same chemicals being used to straighten hair. The future of straightening, however, will be towards less alkaline products, in a similar vein to the acid perm.

8.3 Questions

1   Who originally began the curling of hair?
2   What was the technique devised by wigmakers?
3   How is heat perming different from cold perming?
4   Why was a hook needed when heat perming?
5   Were there any dangers to the client when having such perms?
6   Who was credited with the invention of such perms?
7   What is the croquignole winding method?
8   What is a Callinan perm?
9   What was crêpe hair used for?
10 What was the Jamal system?
11 What does an exothermic sachet do?
12 How is the chemistry of a heat perm different from a cold perm?
13 Why was there a smell of rotten eggs with a heat perm?
14 What is the current trend in perm lotions?
15 Why was a new type of comb needed for black super-curly hair?
16 How was hair first straightened?
17 Why did this method not work for long?
18 What chemical was first used in the 1920s for straightening hair?
19 How have modern straighteners been improved?
20 Why are acid rinses used after straightening?
21 What will be the trend for the future with straighteners?

Glossary

accelerator: a device that produces infra-red radiation as a source of heat to speed up chemical processing of hair, e.g. Climazon.

acid: a chemical compound that contains hydrogen ions, and has a pH of less than 7.0. Acids close the cuticle layer of the hair.

acid conditioners: products which help to reduce oxidation damage and help to restore the hair to its natural pH.

acid wave: a perm product which has a pH reading of between 5.5–7. (See also *true acid wave.*)

activator: any agent that induces activity. In acid perms an activator is mixed with the perm lotion immediately before application to make it work properly.

Afro comb: a comb with widely spaced prongs used for styling and disentangling Afro-type and curly hair.

Afro hair: hair, usually Afro-Caribbean origin, which has a tight curl formation.

albino: a person with no pigment in their hair, skin and eyes.

alkali: a chemical compound that contains hydroxide ions and has a pH of more than 7.0. Alkalis open the cuticle of the hair.

allergy: a reaction to contact with something, usually seen as a change in the skin, which becomes red and inflamed. Not everyone has an allergy, but some hairdressing products recommend a skin test before use on the client to avoid allergic reactions.

alopecia: the term for baldness.

alpha keratin: hair in its unstretched state, hydrogen bonds are intact.

amino acids: the small molecules that proteins are made of; in the cortex they help maintain moisture balance.

ammonium hydroxide: the alkaline chemical that combines with thioglycollic acid to produce ammonium thioglycollate. It is added by manufacturers to cold wave lotions to make them alkaline.

ammonium thioglycollate: the salt which is the active ingredient of most cold wave lotions.

anagen: the active part of the hair growth cycle during which a hair is growing.

analysis: the examination of the client and his or her hair before any hairdressing procedure is carried out. It enables the client to communicate his or her requirements and the hairdresser to carry them out safely without unnecessary damage to the hair.

applicator: an implement (such as a bottle) used to apply a substance to the hair.

arrector pili: the muscle attached to the hair follicle that causes the hair to stand on end on contraction.

artery: a blood vessel that carries blood (usually oxygenated) away from the heart.

backbrushing: brushing back from points to roots to add volume to the hair. Causes the hairs to entangle because the cuticle is damaged.

backwash: a basin in which the client's hair is washed by placing the back of their neck into the basin. It is much safer when using strong chemicals.

baldness: lack of hair in a place where it would be considered normal to have hair.

band marks: lines caused on the hair during perming when the elastic or rubber fastening band of the rod has been incorrectly or too tightly positioned, causing a fracture mark on the hair. This often causes breakage after a perm.

barrier cream: a waterproof cream used to protect the skin from chemicals.

basal layer: the lowest layer of the epidermis where cell division and growth take place (also called the germinating layer).

beta keratin: keratin in its stretched condition.

bonding lotion: an alternative name for *neutraliser.*

breakage: a condition where the hair splits and breaks off. Can be caused by overprocessing or overlapping of chemicals.

buckled ends: this is when a flaw in the winding of the hair around the perm rod causes a frizzy end to the points of the hair. (Also known as *fish hooks.*)

cap: in perming this is a plastic bag which is placed on the client's head to speed up processing by trapping body heat and preventing evaporation of the perm lotion.

cape: a wrap-around protective garment used to protect the clothes of your client.

capillary: the small blood vessels between arteries and veins which supply each hair follicle with blood.

catagen: the stage of the hair growth cycle where the follicle begins to shrink and the hair ceases active growth.

caustic: a strong alkali capable of attacking and damaging other substances. Sodium hydroxide, used in relaxers, is caustic and can severely damage the hair and skin.

chopsticks: straight pieces of wood or plastic used for eating food in Far Eastern countries. In recent years, it has become very popular for hairdressers to use them for perming instead of traditional rods.

citric acid: an organic acid found in citrus fruits, used in neutralisers and acidic rinses to neutralise alkalinity and close the cuticle of the hair.

clip: a clamp-like device used to secure the hair.

clockwise: in hairdressing, the movement of hair in the same direction as the hands of a clock.

coarse hair: a hair fibre with a large diameter.

cold waving: a method of chemically altering the curl of hair without the use of excessive heat.

cold waving lotion: a chemical solution used to alter the bonds in hair so that they can take on another shape, usually containing ammonium thioglycollate.

comb-out: the use of a hair brush or comb to open out hair into the finished style.

concentrated: condensed, usually by the removal of water. Increasing the strength of a chemical solution by decreasing the bulk.

conditioner: any product applied to the hair to improve its condition.

conditioning: the application of special chemicals to the hair to help restore its strength and body.

contra-indications: indications against performing a service.

cortex: the central layer of the hair, consisting of bundles of fibres. Perming and straightening break the disulphide bonds found here.

counter-clockwise: the movement of hair in the opposite direction to the hands of a clock (same as anti-clockwise).

croquignole: winding of the hair from the ends to the scalp.

crown: the top, back part of the head.

curl test: a test performed by the hairdresser at regular intervals during the processing of a perm to determine whether the perm has sufficiently 'taken'.

curler: a circular mould used in perming.

curly perm: (also known as 'curl rearranger'). Chemical applied to hair to remove curl and reform the hair into looser curls in two stages. Often based on ammonium thioglycollate and used on Afro hair.

cuticle: the outer layer of the hair, consisting of several layers of overlapping scales

cyst: a fluid-filled sac that may be found on the head.

cysteic acid: the substance created when hydrogen peroxide reacts with *cystine* (as in over-neutralising).

cysteine: an amino acid containing one sulphur atom. Two cysteines are oxidised to form one cystine molecule during the neutralising process in perming.

cystine: an amino acid containing a disulphide bond, which is reduced by perm lotion to form two cysteine molecules.

damaged hair: hair which is either porous, brittle, split, dry or has little elasticity.

dandruff: overproduction of skin scales, which are seen on the scalp. Also called pityriasis.

decomposition: breaking down of one chemical into two or more other smaller parts.

dense: thick, heavy.

depilatory: chemical agent that will remove hair; perm lotions and straighteners can act as depilatories if left on the hair too long.

dermatitis: inflammation of the skin as the result of being in contact with some external agent, such as perm lotion.

dermis: the layer of the skin below the epidermis.

detergent: an agent that cleanses, a synthetic soap.

disulphide bond: the bond formed between the two sulphur atoms in a molecule of cystine; it is very stable.

dry hair: hair that lacks natural oils (sebum) and moisture.

elasticity: the ability of a hair to be stretched and return to its original length.

elasticity test: a test performed by the hairdresser to assess the strength and condition of the hair's internal structure.

end papers: special papers used to control the ends of the hair in wrapping (winding hair on curlers).

ends: the last few centimetres (one inch) of hair, furthest away from the scalp.

epidermis: the very top layer of the skin; protects the body from physical damage and water loss.

European hair: human hair found on people of European descent; for the purpose of this book reference is made to straight Caucasian hair.

evaporation: when a liquid turns into a gas.

filler: a chemical preparation that equalises porosity by filling in the more porous areas.

fine hair: a hair fibre that is relatively small in diameter.

finger wave: the process of setting the hair in a pattern of waves through the use of fingers, comb and waving lotion.

fish hook: a flaw in the curling of hair that results in the tip ends of hair bending in a direction other than that of the rest of the curl.

foil: a thin sheet of metal, usually aluminium or tin.

follicle: the pit in the skin from which a hair grows.

folliculitis: infection of the hair follicle by bacteria.

fragilitis crinium: alternative name for split ends, a condition caused by harsh treatment. The only remedy is to remove the split ends by cutting.

frizz: hair having too much curl.

hairline: the edge of the scalp where the hair begins.

hair shaft: that part of the hair that projects from the skin.

hair straightener: a chemical that breaks the bonds of the hair enabling curly hair to be made straight.

hard press: achieved by a second pressing on soft-pressed hair (see *soft press*). Gives a better, though still temporary result.

hard water: water that contains calcium and magnesium salts, which will not easily form a lather with soap.

henna: a natural hair dye that can coat the hair and join with sulphur bonds in the cortex, so much so that perming may be adversely affected.

hydrogen peroxide: an oxidising agent used in hairdressing, found in many neutralisers.

hygroscopic: ability of something (such as hair) to absorb moisture from the atmosphere.

imbrications of hair: the points where cuticle scales overlap.

incompatible: two products are said to be incompatible when the presence of one causes the other to react differently than intended.

incompatibility test: a test to determine whether damage would be caused to the hair by the use of a product containing hydrogen peroxide.

infectious: something that can be caught, or passed from one client to the next.

infestation: the invasion of the body surface by small animal parasites such as head lice.

inflammation: the reaction of the body to irritation, usually seen as an area of redness.

infra-red: a type of radiation, which is invisible and gives off heat.

insulation: the process of helping to reduce the passage and loss of heat; during perming, a perm cap acts as an insulator.

ion: an atom or group of atoms which carry an electric charge, due to the gaining or losing of electrons.

keratin: the protein from which hair, skin and nails are made.

kinky: very curly hair.

lanolin: purified sheep's sebum.

lanugo: the fine hair which covers most of the body before birth.

litmus: an indicator of either acidity (red) or alkalinity (blue), available as a liquid or as paper.

Mad Mats: bendable, flat, cloth-covered templates which can be used in a variety of ways in fashion perming.

Marcel waving: a technique of forming waves in the hair by means of heated irons.

massage: manipulation of the scalp or body by rubbing, kneading, stroking or tapping, to increase circulation.

medulla: the air space found in the centre of most hairs.

melanin: the black or brown pigment found in both hair and skin.

melanocytes: the cells which produce the pigment melanin, found in the germinating layer of the epidermis.

mesh: a mesh is formed when the section is divided up for winding; it is usually the width of the main section.

metallic dye: a dye which contains metallic salts, usually referred to as hair colour restorer because it darkens the hair progressively as it is applied.

mitosis: the type of cell division where one cell splits into two and makes an exact copy of itself. It is seen in the growth of both skin and hair.

Molton Permers: flexible foam rods used for perming, also known as Molton Browners.

monilethrix: a condition of the hair which results in the hair being beaded.

nape: the name used to describe the back of the head.

neutral: having neither an acid nor an alkaline pH.

neutralisation: the correct chemical definition refers to the reaction between an acid and an alkali to give a salt and water solution with a neutral pH. In hairdressing it is used for the second oxidation stage of perming, or for returning the hair to an acid pH after relaxing hair.

neutraliser: in hairdressing this refers to the oxidising agent used in the second stage of perming.

neutralising shampoo: the acidic shampoo used after relaxing hair to restore the natural acidity of the hair.

nit: the egg of a head louse, usually found attached to the hair within 1 cm of the scalp.

normalising: an alternative term used in hairdressing for neutralising or the second stage of perming.

occipital: the name of the bone which forms the back of the head.

organic: a substance which contains carbon, derived from living or once living sources.

ortho cortex: a type of cortex only present in Afro-type hair. (See also *para cortex.*)

overlap: when a chemical is applied to new untreated hair and there is an area of crossover with previously treated hair. This is referred to as overlapping. The overlap area may break.

over-processing: over-exposure of hair to chemicals, usually caused by using chemicals which were too strong or by leaving them on too long.

oxidation: the process of adding oxygen or taking away hydrogen, seen in perming and some forms of straightening.

oxidising agent: a chemical which releases oxygen.

papilla: the source of hair growth, found at the base of the hair follicle.

para cortex: a type of cortex only present in Afro-type hair.

pediculosis capitis: the correct name for an infestation caused by head lice.

permanent wave: a wave produced in hair by breaking the disulphide bonds of the cortex with a chemical lotion and reforming them while the hair is on curlers.

pH (potential of hydrogen): the symbol for hydrogen ion concentration; a scale of numbers which tells you exactly how acid or alkaline something is.

pheomelanin: the natural hair pigment responsible for the yellow and red tones in hair.

pin curl: a strand of hairs organised into a flat ribbon form, and wound into a series of continuous untwisted circles within circles.

pityriasis: the correct name for dandruff, the overproduction of epidermal scales.

plastic cap: a cap used during perming to help retain moisture and body heat, and so speed up processing.

porosity: the ability of the hair to absorb liquids.

porosity test: a test to check the porosity of the hair and the condition of the cuticle.

porous: full of pores, able to absorb liquids.

post-damping: applying the perm lotion to the hair once it has been wound.

pre-damping: applying the perm lotion to the hair as the hair is wound.

pre-perm lotion: a product that is applied before perming to help equalise the hair's porosity.

pre-perm test: test to see what perm remains in the hair from previous services.

pressing: a method of straightening kinky hair with a heated iron or comb.

processing time: the period of time required for a chemical action upon the hair to achieve the desired result.

psoriasis: a non-infectious skin condition that is sometimes seen on the scalp, characterised by thick silvery scales.

pull-burn: a burn caused by the perm lotion entering the follicle, because the curler has been wound too tightly.

reduction: the addition of hydrogen or the taking away of oxygen from a compound.

relaxer: a chemical product applied to hair to remove the natural curl.

retouch: the application of hair straightener to a new growth of hair.

rod: another name for curler, referring to round cylinders of varying diameters and lengths.

sebaceous glands: the oil glands attached to the hair follicle; they secrete sebum directly into the hair follicle.

sebum: the oily secretion of the sebaceous gland; helps lubricate and waterproof the skin.

sectioning: dividing the hair into separate parts, or panels.

sectioning clip: a clip used to secure sections of hair.

sensitivity: being easily affected by chemicals, resulting in a skin reaction.

shampoo: to wash the hair with detergent and water; the name given to a soapless detergent used to clean the hair.

soapless shampoo: a shampoo that contains a synthetic detergent rather than a soap. Almost every shampoo used today is soapless.

sodium hydroxide: a caustic chemical, commonly called lye, used in a number of hair relaxers. It can also be used to dissolve hair in blocked basins and drains.

soft press: using a hot comb or hot irons to temporarily straighten curly hair. A soft press differs from a hard press in that it removes less of the curl from the hair because the pressing implement is taken through the hair only once.

spiral winding: winding the hair on a curler from roots to points.

split ends: damage to the ends of the hair which results in splitting along the length of the hair; correct term is *fragilitis crinium*.

spongy: porous.

static electricity: the term used to describe the build-up of a charge on the hair, caused by friction when brushing or combing hair, especially when newly dried.

steamer: a machine used to produce moist, moving heat.

straightener: a chemical product applied to hair to remove curl.

strand test: when used correctly this term should be restricted to the test to see whether a colour result is what is desired, on a few hairs rather than the whole head. In hairdressing, however, it is often used to refer to any test on the hair prior to chemical treatment.

sulphur bonds: bonds found in the cortex which are broken down during perming and relaxing treatments.

tail comb: a comb, half of which is shaped into a slender, tail-like end.

technique: a method of accomplishing a desired aim.

telogen: the resting stage of the growth cycle, prior to anagen beginning again.

tension: stress caused by stretching or firmness in winding.

tepid: neither hot nor cold, lukewarm.

terminal hair: the coarse hair found on the scalp and other areas of the body after puberty (beard, underarms and pubic region).

test curl: a test performed before a permanent wave to help the hairdresser judge the strength of lotion to be used, the ideal rod size and approximate processing time. Sometimes, the result of this test may mean that the hairdresser will advise the client against having a perm at all.

thio: a shortened term used for ammonium thioglycollate.

transparent: allows all light to pass through.

translucent: allows some, but not all, light to pass through.

trichorrhexis nodosa: name given to severely damaged hair caused by physical and/or chemical abuse. This condition is recognised by the swellings along the hair shaft where the hair splits and breaks.

true acid wave: an acid perm where the pH remains below 7 throughout the whole process. Many so-called acid perms become alkaline when the components are mixed together.

ultra-violet: the invisible rays present in sunlight that promote tanning of the skin.

under-processed: insufficient action of chemicals on the hair, such that the desired end result is not achieved. Due to insufficient processing time or the use of too weak a chemical.

Vaseline: a trade mark for petrolatum; a neutral substance often used to protect the scalp.

vein: blood vessel that takes blood back toward the heart.

vellus hair: the soft downy hair found on the body.

vertex: the top, or crown, of the head.

virgin hair: hair which has not been previously chemically processed.

Index

acid perm, 11, 84–9
acids, 10–12
activators, 65, 67, 84
airboy, 68–9, 80–84
air oxidation, 77
alkalis, 10–12
alpha-keratin, 4, 20
amino acids, 4–7
ammonium hydroxide, 72
ammonium thioglycollate, 72–5, 121
analysis, 39–50
androgens, 1

basing, 58
beta-keratin, 4, 20
breakage, 106–7, 108–9
brick wind, 141–3

Callinan machine, 173–4
chemical designing, 128–9
chemical treatment, 19–20
chopstick perm, 165–7
client comfort, 54
Climazon, 69
cold permanent waving, 72–6, 77–9
cortex, 3–5, 7–8, 15–16
croquignole, 172
curl test, 32–3
curler size, 44
curly hair, 12–16
curly perm, 97–103
cuticle, 2–5
cyclical theory, 13–16
cysteine, 72–5, 98–100
cystine, 72–5, 98–100
cysts, 40

dandruff *see* pityriasis

density, 41
dermatitis, 34
diluting perms, 65–6
directional wind, 143–4
discoloration, 107, 111
disulphide bonds, 6, 72–5, 98–100, 114–15,
    124–5, 175–6

elasticity, 25–7, 30
end papers, 64
exothermic sachets, 174

fashion techniques, 132–68
fish-hooks, 107, 110
foam perm, 79–84
follicle, 2
frizz, 105–6

hair, 2–7, 40–43
hard press, 116–18
heat perming, 169–77
henna, 45
herringbone wind, 147–9
history, 169–79
hood drier, 67–8
hydrogen bond, 6–7
hydrolysis, 115, 124–5, 176

incompatibility test, 20–22
infectious conditions, 40

Jamal system, 174
Jetting, 93–7

keratin, 1, 4

lanthionine, 124–5, 175–6
lanugo, 1